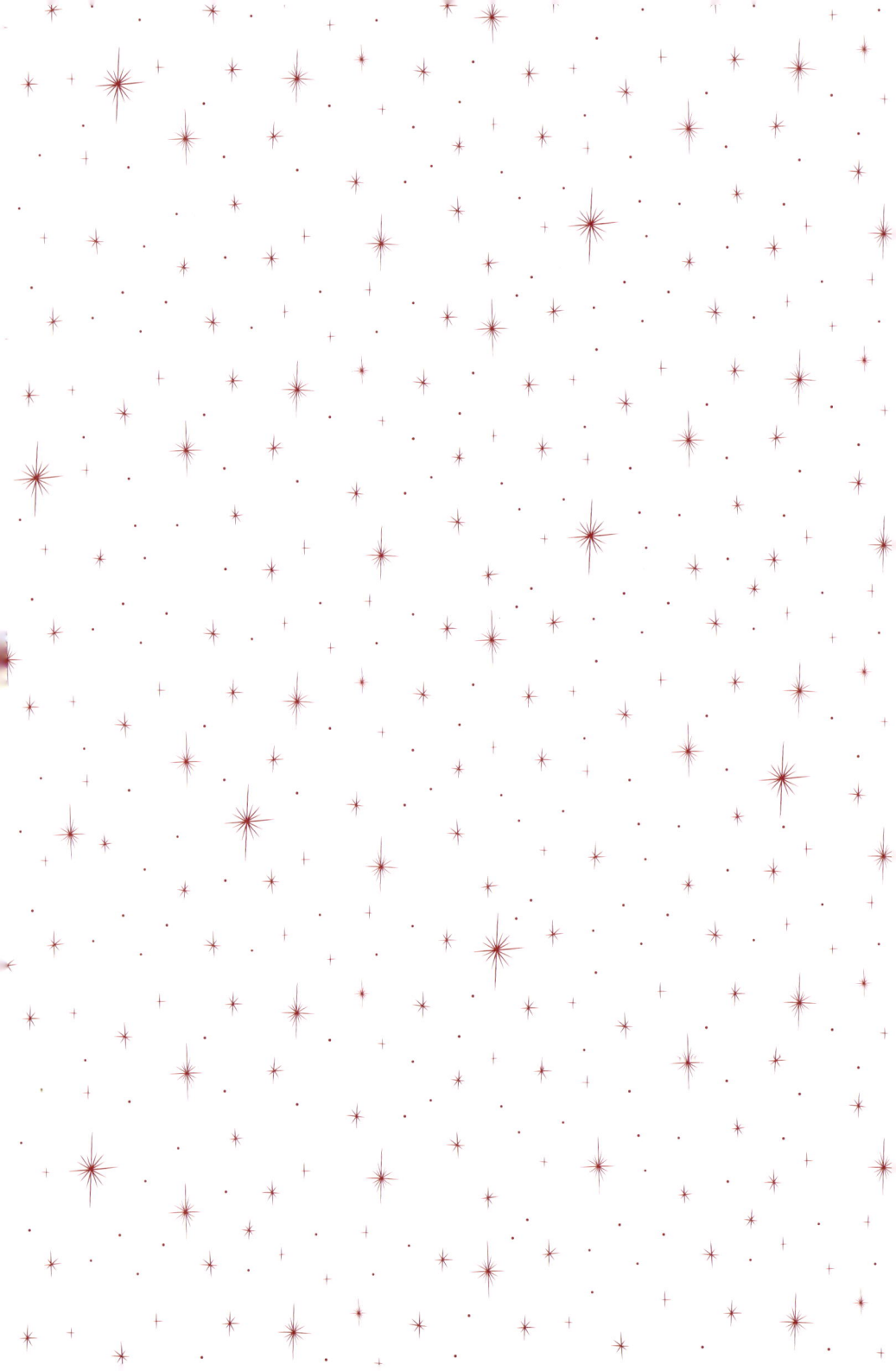

Hormone Goddess

Samantha Hadadi

How to live in harmony with your cycle

VERBENA

Dedication

This book is for Amir and my boys. Who have listened to and supported me through years of talking about the menstrual cycle and the power of women. Who carry the torch for men and boys, and who know that they become stronger when they treasure and cherish the feminine.

It's also for my sisters from other mothers: the women who lift me up, support me, allow me to cry – and who help me to feel unstoppable. To all the women who support me in my work: I love you.

Thank you, too, to my dear friends Em, Rocsi, and Sam. These warm and radiant women are some of the most powerful healers I know. Each has the most incredible knowledge to help women on their journeys, and I am honoured that they have all helped me in some way in this book. I cannot thank them enough.

And finally, for all my ancestors, for my family, who have supported and lifted me, overcome their own stories, bared their own wounds, and walked their own paths to get me here: thank you.

Dear Goddesses,

Thank you for picking up this book. As you turn these pages, I hope that you feel enveloped with love, sisterhood, and understanding.

See this book as your very own permission slip, written to you from me. See it as permission to rest and restore, or as permission to start loving your body, and recognising that you deserve so much more.

As you read on, I hope that you'll start to feel more confident when it comes to advocating for yourself.

This book isn't designed to be taken in place of medical advice. Instead, it's a loving nudge to help you to feel empowered enough that you will never be dismissed or unheard. You don't deserve to be on this journey alone.

With love from me to you,

Sam xxx

Safety note

While I do offer some nutrition advice in this book, please be aware that some women who have allergies, or are pregnant, or have underlying health conditions, may need to take care when it comes to eating certain foods. If you are unsure, always speak to your doctor, or a qualified nutritional therapist for advice.

Contents

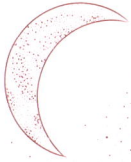

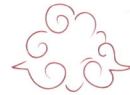

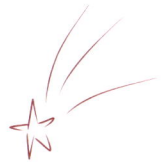

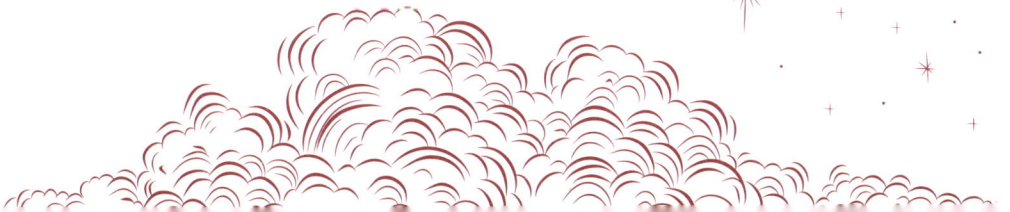

It's not your fault

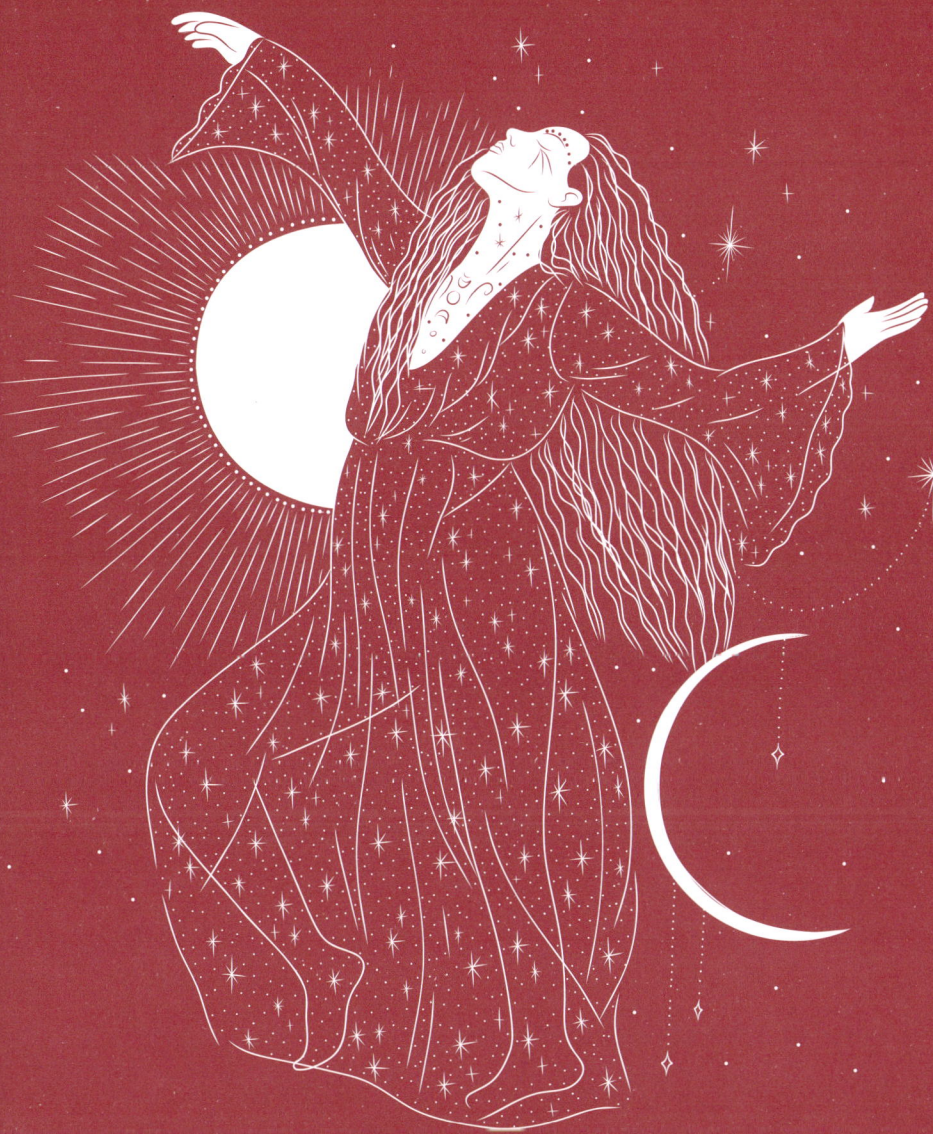

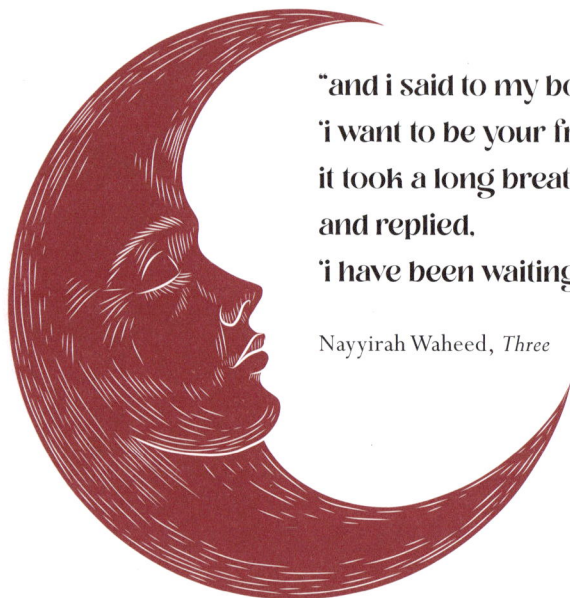

"and i said to my body, softly,
'i want to be your friend.'
it took a long breath,
and replied,
'i have been waiting my whole life for this.'"

Nayyirah Waheed, *Three*

We all deserve to live a "life extraordinary". A life that's full of joy, purpose, and love. A life that comes in technicolour. As women, we also deserve to feel powerful, untamed, and uncaged – wolverines running wild and free across a lush landscape, ready to chase and follow our dreams.

And yet, almost all women I speak to – and perhaps you too – are unable to do this.

Instead, they feel as though they're tethered and trapped. They're in pain, burned out, and suffering with their periods, perimenopause, or countless symptoms triggered by wayward hormones. Most months they struggle with debilitating PMS, tender breasts, and chronic bloating. Mood changes that swing from red-hot rage to teary and anxious at breakneck speed. Yet, alongside this, there's a common thread that entwines us all: we don't realise that we no longer need or deserve to struggle, or even that there's another way. This is because most women (me included) have been taught that period problems, and chronic pain and suffering, are part of the pink ribbon that ties up our experience of womanhood.

This book is here to tell you it's not.

Because, no matter what you've been told, it's not normal.

It's not normal to live in pain, to have breasts so sore you can't exercise, or mood swings so severe they give you whiplash.

It's not normal to struggle with your menstrual cycle and hormones – and it most definitely isn't your fault if you do.

Goddess, I'm so glad you're here, and I'm so glad that you have this book in your hands. It's time to make friends with your hormones and your body, because you deserve so much more.

The Truth

So, if you take just one thing from this book, make it this: suffering with your cycle is not normal. In fact, here's a list of all the things that are not normal, and that you shouldn't have to put up with just "because you're a woman":

· Heavy or painful periods

· Passing large clots

· Frequent digestive issues

· Brain fog

· Persistent fatigue

· Severe mood swings

· Anxiety or depression

· Thinning hair

· Acne

· Unexplained weight gain

I could go on, because there are endless symptoms related to our hormones. Yet, hopefully you'll come to see as you read this book, you don't need to suffer.

We'll learn more as we go, but each one of these signs and symptoms can point to hormonal imbalances or underlying conditions. They can also signal emotional wounds that need healing – love that needs giving, memories that need releasing and beliefs that need challenging. It's difficult to recognise this when you're in the midst of crippling cramps, or you've just flooded through a super plus tampon and pad in the middle of the supermarket. Yet, symptoms are the body's language, guiding you back to love.

However much you're struggling, however much pain you're in, I promise that you can restore harmony.

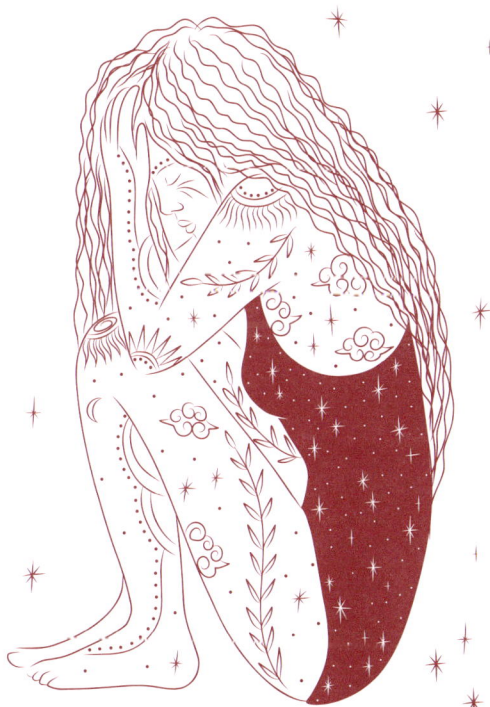

You're Not Alone

When I first started learning about my hormones, I felt alone. I'd wander down the street and look mournfully at all the women whom I thought were living their best lives.

I'd stare enviously at the taut yoga bodies (I struggled endlessly with weight gain), or feel frustrated as I spied glamorous women in power suits, tapping furiously away on their phones (my own brain fog meant I couldn't function past 1pm, let alone be a "success").

I'd also feel deep shame about the way I looked. I would slather on trowels-full of make-up to cover my acne and fatigue, before desperately scouring my wardrobe for clothes that would skim over the parts of my body I loathed.

I felt isolated.

I believed that I was the only one struggling, and that all other women were living a perfect, radiant, joyful life.

Of course, this wasn't true – a quick Google search now tells me that 80–90% of women struggle with hormonal health at some point in their lives. A staggering 84% feel as though their healthcare providers don't always listen to them.

One day, the world needs to be different for our daughters and granddaughters. Yet, for now, whatever symptoms you may or may not have, please know that you're not alone. Wherever you are on your journey, you're enveloped in love, understanding, and sisterhood.

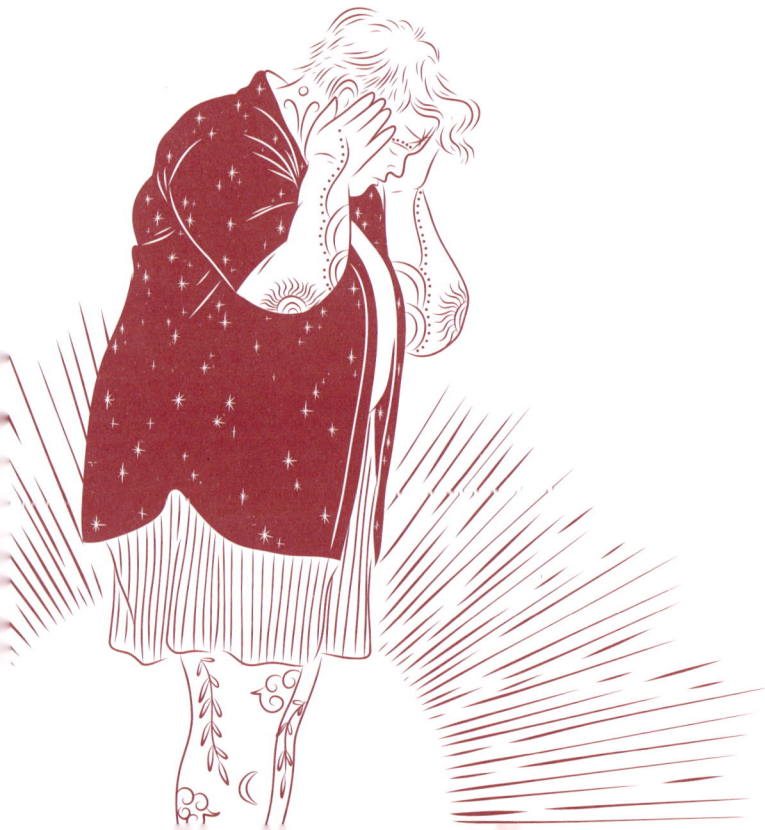

Just Like You

We all know women who have tales to tell and horror stories to share about their periods. Perhaps that woman is you.

As you've seen, for most of my life I was much the same – I loathed getting my period and, frankly, I hated being a woman. I grimaced when that first flush of crimson appeared in my knickers each month. I knew that it meant I was in for a whirlwind of pain, fatigue, dizziness, and swollen, cyst-like acne. Each month, I'd feel like I was losing my mind as hot, angry rage bubbled up inside. I'd swallow it down (because, let's face it, when are women encouraged to be angry?), only for it to explode out of me.

I'd then feel sticky with shame, as though I were broken.

And then, of course, there was the bleeding itself. I'd have to crawl to the toilet, scared of flooding my pads and bleeding onto our new carpet. I'd swallow down pills to mask the pain, then glower and simmer and curse being a woman, as I tried my best to pretend my body wasn't there. As you'll read in the next chapter, my hormones threw me into the depths of despair. I almost drowned. Yet, it led me here, where I now get to help other women to understand and cherish their bodies. So, I write this book to you from the deepest place of love.

As I sit at my desk, surrounded by peace lilies and snake plants, and with a steaming mug of cacao nestled in my lap, I can tell you that you're not broken. That you can live a life free from pain and the dreaded "monthly curse".

Heck, you can even learn to love your period!

When you follow the juicy tips and tricks I'm going to share with you in this book – and, more importantly, when you follow your own wisdom – your menstrual cycle will become your superpower. It will become your spark, your inner guidance system, your creativity, and your magic, all bundled up in one. It's part of what makes you *you*.

Of course, it can be difficult to tap into this when we live in pain, and when we associate our bodies with suffering. And that is what this book is here for, to erase the shame that you may feel goes hand-in-hand with womanhood.

Hand on heart, I can honestly say that I *love* being a woman. And no matter your starting point, you can too.

Questioning the "Norm"

Perhaps it's my inner rebellious streak, or perhaps it's simply down to the fact that I'm a dreamer; yet one thing I never really got was why women have to suffer with their periods.

Why, when half of the population is born female, have we never questioned why we're meant to just grin and bear it?

Why, when we talk about our period struggles, are we so often dismissed with a hasty prescription for the pill?

And why, with all the medical advances, do we need to accept that suffering is tethered to womanhood?

The answer is more complex than this book can ever go into. In fact, it deserves a whole book entirely of its own. For example, did you know that erectile dysfunction is studied and researched *five* times more than PMS? This is in spite of the fact that the majority of women suffer with PMS at some point in their lives, while just 19% of men struggle with erectile dysfunction. Try reading that and *not* feeling righteous, feminine rage.

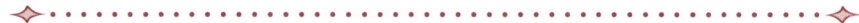

Education, Education, Education

For many of us though, I've come to realise that much of the problem lies in what we don't know. Or, more accurately, what we haven't been taught.

In other words, it's not your fault.

What often goes hand-in-hand with our menstrual cycles is a lack of awareness about our beautiful bodies. This runs through healthcare, but it's also etched into the bones of the school system. Whichever way we spin it, sex education is – for the most part – woefully lacking. Unless you were one of the lucky few, you were likely taught just the bare basics of biology, or how not to get pregnant and catch an STD.

Chances are, you weren't even taught simple anatomy. How many of us speak about the vagina when we really mean the vulva, for example? How many of us know the difference between the labia minora and the labia majora, or what the cervix actually does?

If you don't... don't feel shame. I didn't know until my mid-thirties!

One of the only memories I have of my sex education was sitting, aghast, as the teacher gleefully – sadistically – told us how much pain our periods could bring. She then dangled around a few tampons and whipped out a few stray pads, before wheeling out the ancient TV set and hitting play on a video.

In all honesty, I don't remember much else beyond the fear-based: "you're going to bleed, and it's going to be hell". As a result, I could barely tell my mum or my Nanna when I got my first period. I felt as though I would die with shame when I had to buy myself tampons or pads in shops, or when a friend dared to bring up their period.

It's likely the story holds true for you, too. Very few of us are taught about the magic of our cycles. Instead, we're taught about "sanitary towels" or "feminine hygiene", as though our bodies are inherently dirty. We're told to keep our periods "hush-hush", or to stash our tampons up our sleeves rather than admit to the world that we are bleeding. I also have to mention that we live in a society where – whichever way you spin it – women are overly sexualised or criticised. If we don't look like glossy, long-legged, shiny-haired supermodels (and even if we do), we're made to feel lesser. We're manipulated and prodded into hiding and transforming and starving our bodies, and this pressure only grows as we age. From a young age, we're taught we should cover ourselves up, lest we tempt men. If we don't shun short skirts, or if we refuse to wear polo necks to cover our breasts, we're provocative, or "asking for it". Of course, there are no winners here – even if we do cover up we're labelled "frumpy" or unattractive.

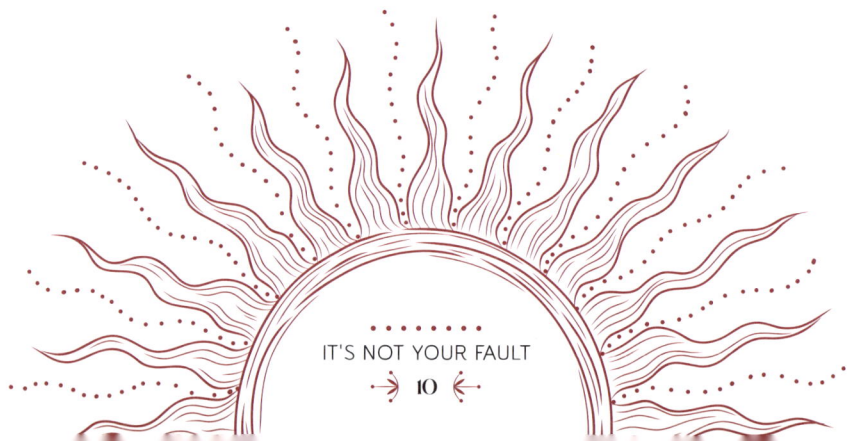

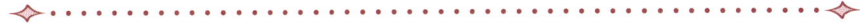

The point is, that no matter what we do, our periods — and our bodies — become entwined with misery and pain.

For many women, I believe that this is where our struggles start: with our education (or lack of it), and the messages we're taught. Our emotions aren't separate from our biology, and we internalise these beliefs and hold onto them as stress. Eventually, it becomes our experience of womanhood.

As you'll come to see, ready-packaged shame can become hormonal imbalance, PMS, and painful periods. Unresolved trauma, chronic stress, and poisonous thoughts can all impact our beautiful bodies, particularly the HPA axis (hypothalamic-pituitary-adrenal axis), which helps us to cope with stress.

These things can also disrupt the delicate balance of female hormones, such as progesterone and oestrogen, and can wreak havoc with insulin, our thyroid, and androgen levels. As well as this, our womb spaces and pelvic bowls are like chalices. They hold our stories, our journeys, and our emotions, as well as our traumas and our ancestral pain.

In other words, what the mind suppresses, the womb expresses.

If you want to dig deeper, and if you want to heal your hormones, you need to start considering what beliefs you've been taught to hold onto. The beliefs that really aren't your fault.

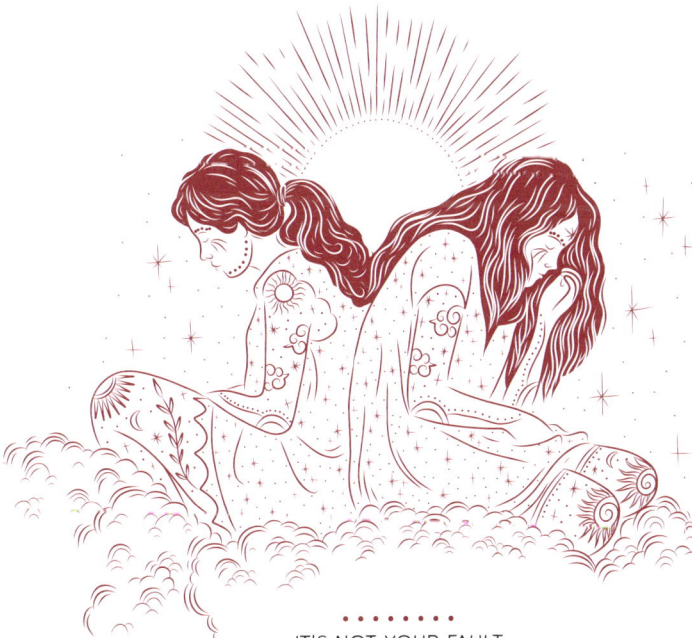

The Medical World

Unfortunately, when we don't understand our bodies, it becomes easy to revert back to default mode: to ignore the aches and pains, and to simply swallow a pill so we can get on with life. When we aren't given the education we deserve, we have no idea what we are meant to feel like and what our bodies are truly capable of.

And this leads me onto the next reason why women like you and I have such a struggle and a fight on our hands: the medical world is (for the most part) stacked against us.

While many doctors are doing their best in an under-funded, over-stressed environment, many of us have jaded and traumatic experiences. All too often, we're dismissed. In the case of women struggling with debilitating conditions such as endometriosis or PCOS (polycystic ovary syndrome), we might wait years and years (a diagnosis for endometriosis in the UK now takes an average of nine years) for the help we deserve.

I've heard countless stories of women having the coil fitted, screaming and writhing in agony. I've heard of women collapsing on the floor in hospital emergency departments in debilitating pain, only to be sent home with a prescription for paracetamol.

Until 1993, women of "child-bearing age" didn't even have to be part of medical and health trials in the United States. This was, in part, due to the fact that there was fear surrounding what untested medications could do to unborn babies (partly a result of the thalidomide tragedy). The implication here is that we are valued solely on our capacity to reproduce. Yet, there were also those who believed women were simply "mini men", and that therefore there was no need to test on both sexes, because there was no difference between them anyway.

As a result, women continue to be under-represented in medical care. Certain drugs are prescribed using dosages which have been based on male physiology. Women continue to be misdiagnosed when they have heart disease (studies show that women may be 50% more likely to be misdiagnosed than men), or sent home from emergency departments when they're having heart attacks. Why? Because their symptoms can sometimes differ from men's, whom the research was based on.

I don't know about you, but this makes my blood boil!

Because when it comes to our pain and suffering, women are not always taken seriously. And if we're lucky? Many women and girls who – like me – visit their doctor in pain, or with heavy bleeding or acne, are merely dismissed with a slip of paper for the pill.

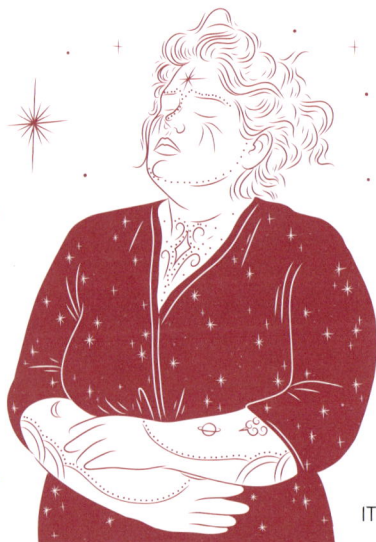

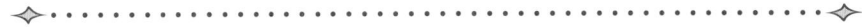

The Pill

The birth control pill first became available in 1961, with the promise of liberating women and paving the way for us to enjoy our sexuality. Yet, in the years that followed, the pill became a one-stop shop. It was used for preventing unwanted pregnancies, but it was also prescribed for painful periods, heavy bleeding, acne, and so much more. The problem occurs when the pill is handed over without exploring the root cause of a woman's symptoms. When used this way, it becomes a sticking plaster, masking our symptoms without addressing the root cause.

For many women – me included – the birth control pill also makes symptoms worse over time.

Whatever your view – and this isn't me telling you to quit the pill (we all have to do what's right for our own bodies!) – it's important to understand that the pill will never work to balance your hormones, nor will it ever treat your symptoms. Many women are also not given the full picture. Did you know that a pill bleed isn't a real period, for example? Instead, it's a withdrawal bleed and occurs when the artificial hormones are stopped. To help you to be prepared, and to help you talk to your doctor with more awareness and understanding, here are just a few of the potential side-effects of taking the pill:

· The pill can impact gut health (which, ultimately, is crucial for hormone health).

· It can deplete us of certain nutrients and vitamins, including magnesium, selenium, zinc, B vitamins, and vitamins C and E.

· It can impact testosterone levels and libido, meaning we miss out on years of great sex.

· Pills that suppress ovulation mean we are missing out on a natural balance of hormones, which are crucial for a woman's health.

· It can affect the HPA axis and how our bodies are able to deal with, and respond to, stress.

Incredibly, the pill can even impact who we are attracted to. This means that you could even fall for the wrong person while taking it! Taking the pill can also mean we feel out of touch with our bodies. By taking synthetic hormones, we have no idea of our feminine magic. We don't understand those natural shifts, changes, and super powers – and we have no idea what we are capable of.

Hopefully by now, you're starting to see that the problem is deep-rooted and multi-layered. But if you're struggling, please know this: it is not your fault.

Monthly Report Cards

It's not all doom and gloom in the medical world, though – and change is afoot.

More and more, it's becoming recognised that our periods are a reflection of our health. In other words, your doctor should be helping you to see your menstrual cycle as your very own monthly report card.

Our cycles are now known as one of the vital signs of health. Along with other crucial measures of health, such as body temperature, pulse rate, and respiration rate, our periods are seen as a mirror of our overall health, habits, and lifestyle. So, if you ever need to speak to a doctor about your periods, now you know: your suffering is far from normal, and it deserves to be taken seriously.

Reflection
Ritual

✧ • • • • • • • • • • • • • • • • • • ✧

Before we continue onwards and you learn how to support your body, I encourage you to sit and reflect on your own journey here, to this book. To do this, here are some questions to help you explore any emotional roots of hormonal issues, or underlying beliefs that may be impacting your biology.

To answer these questions, find yourself a pen and paper, some stillness and take a few deep breaths. When you're ready, free write (write without preconception), and see what comes up. Whatever the answers you write, try to view them without judgement.

· What were you taught about your periods when you were younger?

· What was your first bleed like? How did it feel?

· When you started your period, did you understand what was happening? Did you feel supported and held, or were you scared, fearful, or ashamed?

· How might these experiences have impacted your cycle, or your relationship with your body?

· If your first bleed had been celebrated, how might your relationship with your cycle be different now?

· What did your younger self need to be taught so you could thrive?

· How do you currently view your periods and your cycle?

· How do you feel towards your body?

· Do you enjoy being a woman?

· How do you feel when you get your bleed?

· What do you do when you get your period? What would you like to do?

· When you hear your friends or other women talking about their periods, how do you feel?

· What has your overall journey with your hormones been like?

· If you've needed to seek help or support for your hormones, what has your experience been like?

· How do you feel about ageing and the next phase of your life (menopause)?

It's Really Not Your Fault

Finally, I want to repeat: it's not your fault.

It's *not your fault*.

It's not your fault if you're struggling, because you've never been shown your period and your beautiful body in the magical light it deserves.

Unfortunately, it can be hard to pass this message on, so please tell your friends, your sisters, your daughters, your granddaughters – we need to spread the word far and wide. Please share it with your sons and male partners, too, because men also need to understand our rhythms.

With this book, we can start imagining a new future, and we can become the change that we all so desperately need and want.

Spread the message far and wide: period pain is not normal, and we do not need to suffer.

Now, from one sister to another, let's sit down and learn all about our beautiful bodies.

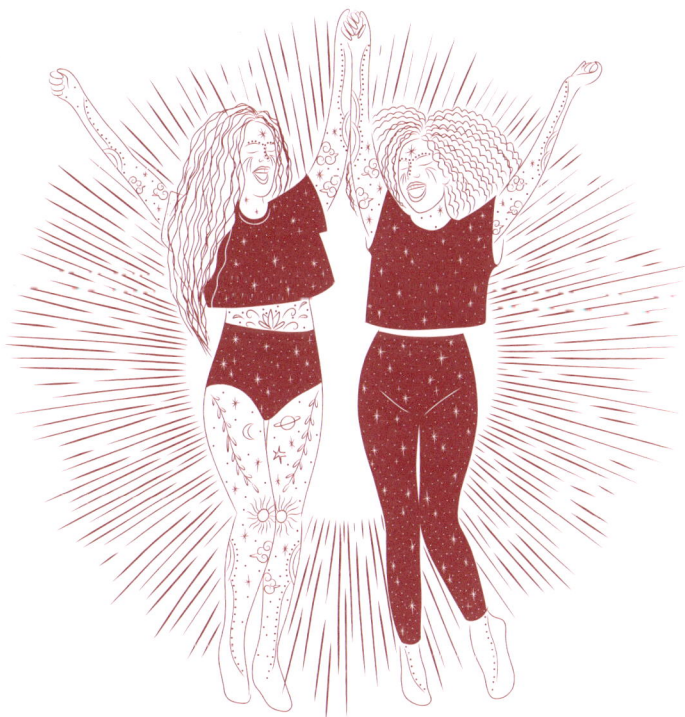

My Journey

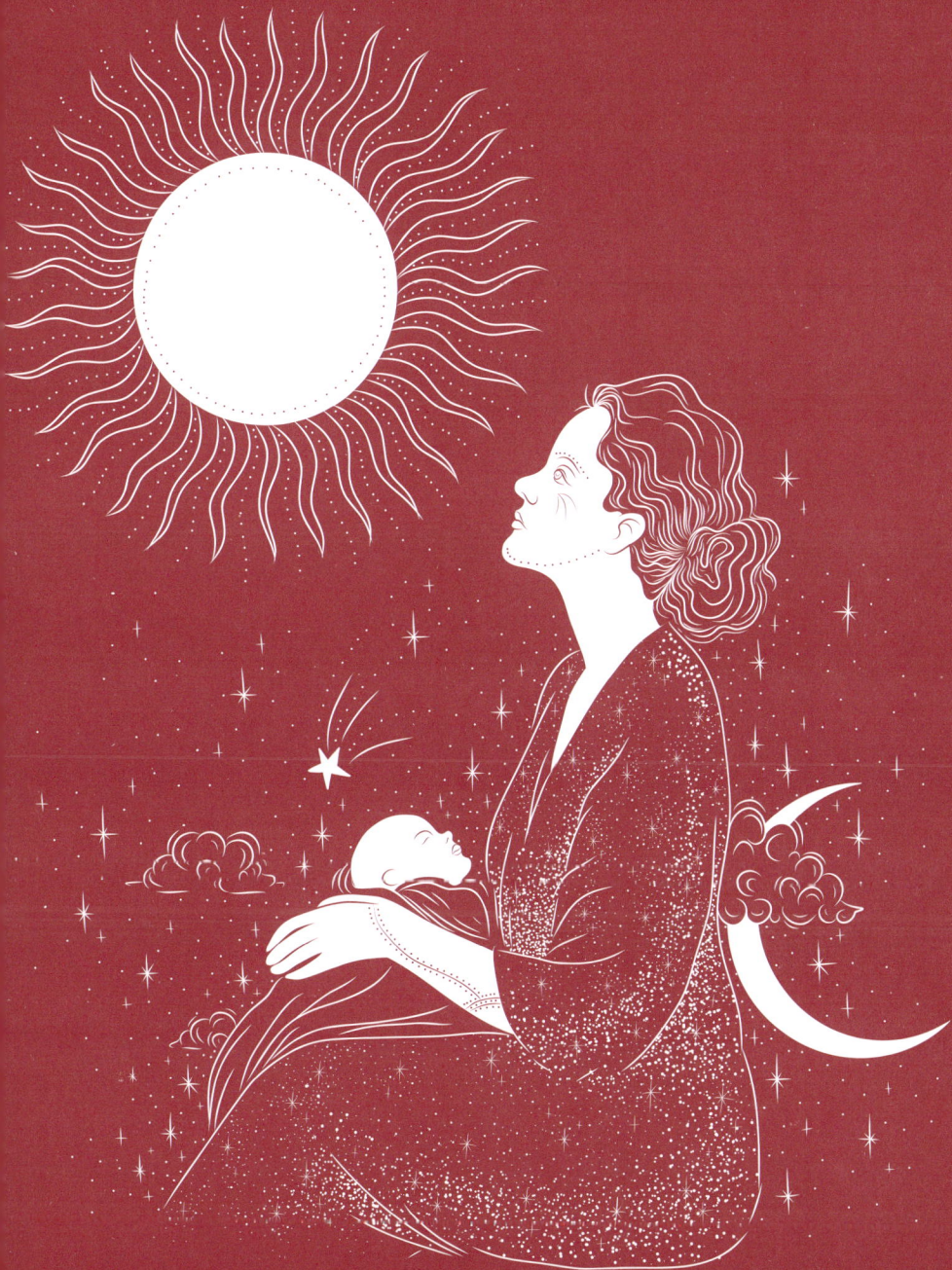

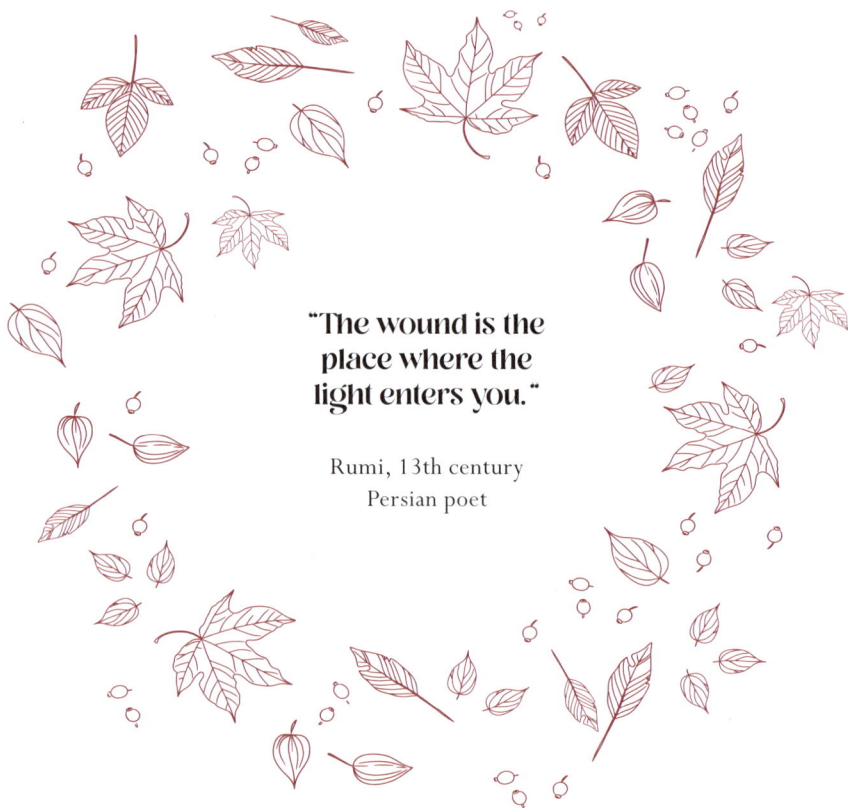

> ## "The wound is the place where the light enters you."
>
> Rumi, 13th century
> Persian poet

It's hard to realise it when you're submerged in darkness, but our shadows can be filled with light. While my past has been traumatic at times (and, likely, so has yours), I'm lucky enough to be in a position now where I can be grateful for it. Ultimately, my story has been my medicine.

Overcoming my traumas is what's led me here — to you, to writing this book, and living out my childhood dreams. But, believe me when I say that my journey has been a rocky one. I didn't always see my period in a positive light, and there have been times when my moods were so bleak and dark that I couldn't see any way out.

If you're reading this and feel as though there's little place for light, please know that you're not alone. But please also seek help and support — you don't have to suffer on your own, and there's always another way.

Here, I'll share a little of my journey in the hope that it helps someone to feel less alone.

My Journey Here

From a young age, I struggled with my body. I was the girl whose breasts budded and bloomed early, whose hips arced and curved into voluptuous silhouettes. It made me painfully, achingly self-conscious. I didn't want to be different. I didn't want to stand out. I just wanted to be like my friends.

And then, I got my period before anyone else that I knew.

From the moment that first petal of red stained my knickers, I felt ashamed of my bleed. I was so embarrassed, so mortified, that I stuffed my underwear with toilet paper and didn't tell anyone for days.

Day one of my entry into womanhood, and the deep hatred towards my cycle had already begun. Perhaps unsurprisingly, I struggled with my hormones from that moment onwards.

My periods were cripplingly heavy and painful. I would flood through my pads and I was put on tablets to stem my bleeding. I'd feel dizzy and sick from heavy blood loss, and I'd be constantly, chronically paranoid that I'd bleed through my clothes at school or during PE. I also had severe acne which made me want to cover and hide my face. I felt constantly sad and tearful, and desperately unlovable.

No one really knew what to do with me. My mum (through no fault of her own) didn't have much knowledge about periods and hormones – a trip to the doctors was the only answer she had. And so, from the age of 13 or 14, I was placed on the pill to stem the tide of my heavy bleeding and to ease my acne. It worked, too! For years, I was able to live (relatively) pain-free, and my skin calmed down. However, the pill also made me numb to my body. It worked to keep me disconnected, oblivious to what was simmering beneath the surface.

When I reached my later teenage years, my cycle of self-loathing only grew. I would pore over magazines, hoping to transform into the look of the tall and lithe supermodels of the 90s. I would stand in front of a mirror, pinching and prodding my skin, willing it to shrink and disappear.

And, of course, I absorbed the toxic messaging that abounded in the 90s and 00s (and, likely, long before I was born). I convinced myself that I was fat and I tried every diet around: Special K, low-fat, low-carb, low-calorie.

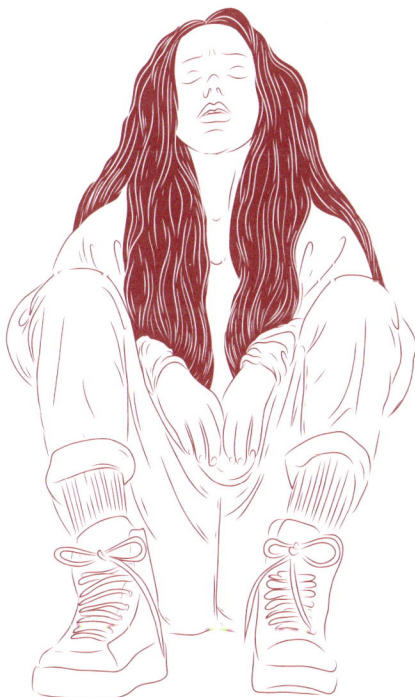

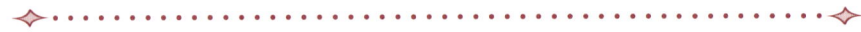

The End, and the New Beginning

In an effort to stifle the pain, I'd become a master at squashing down my emotions by the time I hit my twenties.

Scared of unveiling and sitting with my feelings, I hurtled through life at breakneck speed. I was always busy, always rushing, always doing. I said "yes" to everything and everyone. Jumped at the chance to party, drink, and dance into the early hours. By staying manic, I convinced myself that my life shimmered and shone.

Of course, it was all a facade – and by my late twenties, it came tumbling down. Although, I wasn't to know that just yet.

Fast forward a few years, and I was married and a stay-at-home mum to my beautiful toddler. I was still always busy, still always racing around, and still always seeing people, but I was desperately, achingly lonely.

I had harboured dreams of writing and becoming an author, but they'd been shelved – for now. My husband had a good job, we had a beautiful house, enjoyed fancy holidays, and I had a wardrobe packed with clothes that once I only dreamed of having.

I was also expecting my second boy, Leo, and I loved being pregnant. As I watched my belly start to stretch and swell, and then ripple with tiny kicks and stretches, I felt what it was like to be loved.

From the outside, my life looked perfect. From my own deeply rose-tinted perspective, my life looked perfect. And yet, somewhere buried deep, deep down, a deep rot had set in. Everything was crumbling beneath me.

As I went into my final trimester of pregnancy, I'd find myself unable to sleep. I'd lie awake all night, heart hammering, throat tight and raw, body shaking. I had no idea what was causing the insomnia. I tried everything that I could – lavender, chamomile, hot baths, meditations. Sobbing and crying, I begged my doctor to prescribe sleeping pills – anything to take away this feeling.

Yet, she didn't – she couldn't. And nothing else would shift it.

My lack of sleep continued until I became so tired, so broken, that I felt hollowed out and stripped to the bones. I'd lie awake, sobbing and howling, until sweeps of apricot began to tinge the sky. I'd stumble through my days on a diet of black coffee, dashing between play groups and play dates with my toddler.

I honestly had no idea what was coming.

I had no idea that my insomnia was a sign: that my body knew what my mind didn't, and my life was shifting beneath me.

A week before I was due to give birth to Leo, the foundations collapsed.

My marriage crumbled as I discovered things about my then-husband. Put simply: he was an addict, and he wasn't who I thought he was. Our life wasn't what I thought it was. He'd betrayed me, betrayed the boys, and damaged our family beyond repair. After the police laid the truth bare – my ex couldn't tell me to my face – I realised that none of our life had been real. We were also up to our eyeballs in debt.

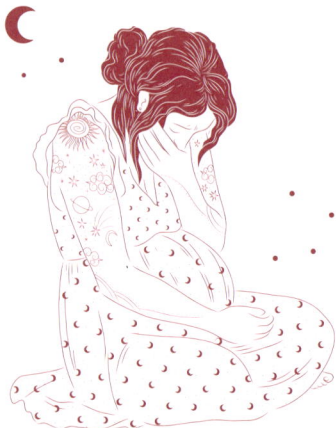

I gave birth in a haze – the midwives had to force-feed me sweets to stop me from falling asleep as I pushed Leo out – and stumbled through those first weeks postpartum.

I still don't remember them, and I don't know if I ever will.

I was forced to start my own business just a week or two after birth. We had no money to pay for our mortgage, and debts to repay – I had little choice. I didn't know what else I could do, so I taught myself food photography and became a recipe developer.

What followed from my ex-husband was lie after lie, chance after chance, and trauma after trauma. As I juggled life with a newborn, a toddler and a burgeoning business, my marriage eroded to the point that there was nothing left. No ruins, nothing to rebuild, and I eventually kicked him out.

It should have been the end of that chapter, and the start of a new one. And yet, it wasn't.

What followed was a stretch of trauma after trauma – endless court battles, harassment from a stalker, a soul-crushing abortion. And then, finally, picking up the shattered pieces after my ex decided he wanted nothing more to do with my – with our – children.

In the midst of this chaos, my partner Amir and I also had my third boy, Ezra.

I had everything thrown at me in those years, so perhaps it doesn't come as a shock that I transformed into a jittering, anxious, sick wreck. I was your "poster woman" for hormonal imbalances: stressed, traumatised, disconnected, pushing myself to the brink.

I survived on coffee, skipping meals here, there and everywhere, and my body teetered dangerously, chaotically, close to the edge. Perhaps you can imagine just how well it went when, in the midst of all this, I suddenly decided I no longer wanted to take the pill.

My periods once again became heavy and painful. I'd stand up and flood through tampons and pads. I'd feel weak, sick and exhausted, and I began to gain weight. My body ballooned and burst from my clothes. My hair thinned and fell out, my hands and feet felt permanently cold, and I had brain fog so thick and murky that I couldn't function past 1pm. I was wracked with anxiety, and saw worst case scenarios about *everything*.

Thankfully, I'd worked as a ghost writer for a nutritionist who specialised in women's health, so I understood that I had a thyroid issue, and I knew about how to eat and nourish my body to help it to heal. Yet, even though I was eating "All The Right Things", something still wasn't quite clicking into place. I was still sick, and still gaining weight – and the weight-gain only grew worse the more exercise I took.

Slowly, I came to realise: my traumas and my health had, somehow, collided. What I had been through had tampered with my hormones.

I felt this in my bones, but no one could tell me how. No one wanted to listen – doctors wanted to put me back on the pill, or insert the copper coil (long story short: that made my symptoms worse than ever). Nutritionists couldn't give me any more of an answer or more of a clue.

So, I decided to learn to navigate my own way.

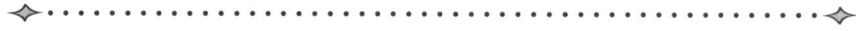

The Next Chapter

Deep in the depths of the COVID pandemic, I trained as a health coach. As Amir and I juggled home schooling our four boys with running our own businesses, I spent a year immersed in a holistic health coaching course.

As I studied, I delved deep into how to support the body using food as medicine. I delved into spirituality, relationships, and our environment – and the effect it could have on health. And I delved into what I had neglected for so long: the need for deep, restorative rest.

At the same time (I don't do things by halves), I studied for a separate coaching qualification in hormone health. I learned more about our hormones and the female anatomy. I prodded and probed and learned about the A-Z of the endocrine system, about the signs of imbalances – and how to heal from them.

I also learned about adrenal fatigue (something which, I came to realise, had impacted me), and the havoc that chronic stress can unleash on your thyroid.

I learned all the things about our hormones (and more) that I wish I'd been taught from a young age, including our cyclical nature – and the importance of living in tune with our cycles.

Slowly, as I started to put into practice all the things I was learning (and, crucially, honouring my need to rest), I began to reassemble my body and my health. My periods became pain-free, and the weight fell off me – no dieting needed. My skin cleared, and my sleep fell into place. My anxiety completely vanished.

Ultimately, I learned what I now teach: our periods and our hormones aren't just a reflection of our physical health, but a reflection of our emotional and spiritual health, too.

Womb Healing

Ever since, I've become fascinated by the role trauma can have on our health and hormones. I went on to train as a somatic teacher so that I can help women to unlock stuck trauma, and I'm also a Womb Priestess, and trained in womb healing.

I was initiated at Glastonbury as a Womb Priestess in 2024. As a priestess, I'm dedicated to helping other women to rediscover the power in their own bodies, heal their traumas, and connect to their divine, feminine light. There are lots of ways I do this, such as shamanic journeying, women's circles, and ceremonies and rituals. However, as a priestess, I try to lead through power and softness – helping women to see the depths of magic that lie within.

As you'll come to learn, our wombs (or our womb spaces, if you don't have a womb) are the centre of a woman's power. They're our life force energy source, where we hold our confidence, creativity, and sexual energy. Yet, when our wombs are filled with trauma or pain, this energy leaks out of us. We feel numb, disconnected, and stuck.

I experienced this myself. As I worked with my own womb, magic began to happen. I was able to unpeel layers of trauma and pain which lay there. The more I unpeeled, the more my body unravelled – and sadness, anger, and sharp pain tumbled out of me.

Sexual trauma, trapped and stagnant emotions, miscarriage and abortion pain, and even my own birth (my mum nearly died when she was having me), all bubbled up to the surface. Working with the womb helped me to heal traumas that no amount of therapy ever could – and my body suddenly came alive.

And now? Well, this is just the beginning of my journey – I'm quite sure that there's much more to come.

But, I'm here because I've been where you are, too. And I want to help you clear the fog, to find your way – because you know, deep down, that you deserve better.

Deep down, you know there's another way.

Deep down, you know you're not meant to suffer.

And I'm here to support you through it.

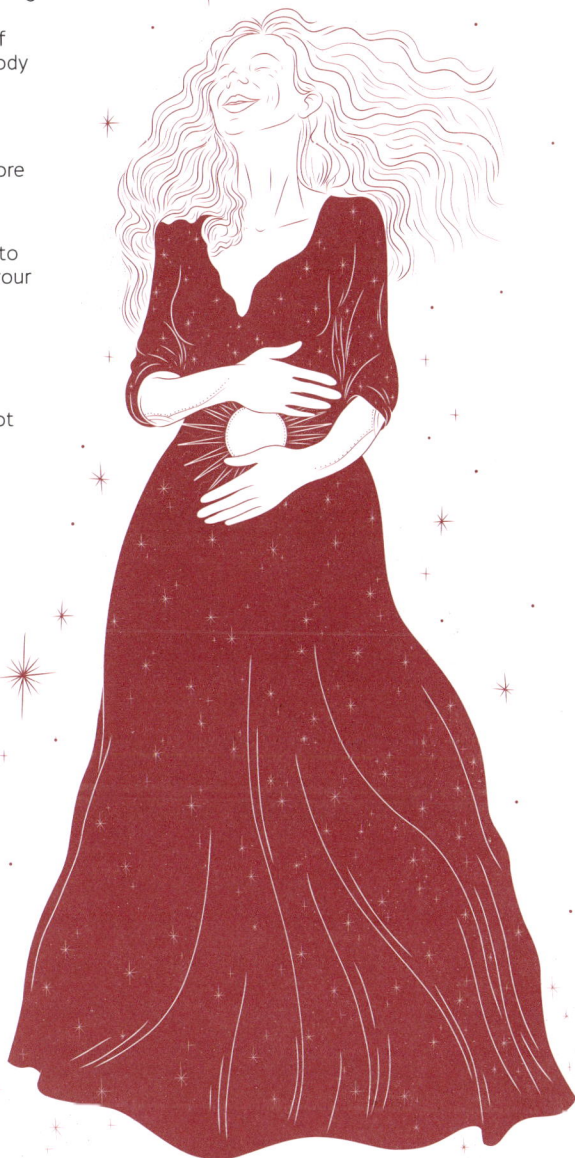

Your Cycle is Sacred

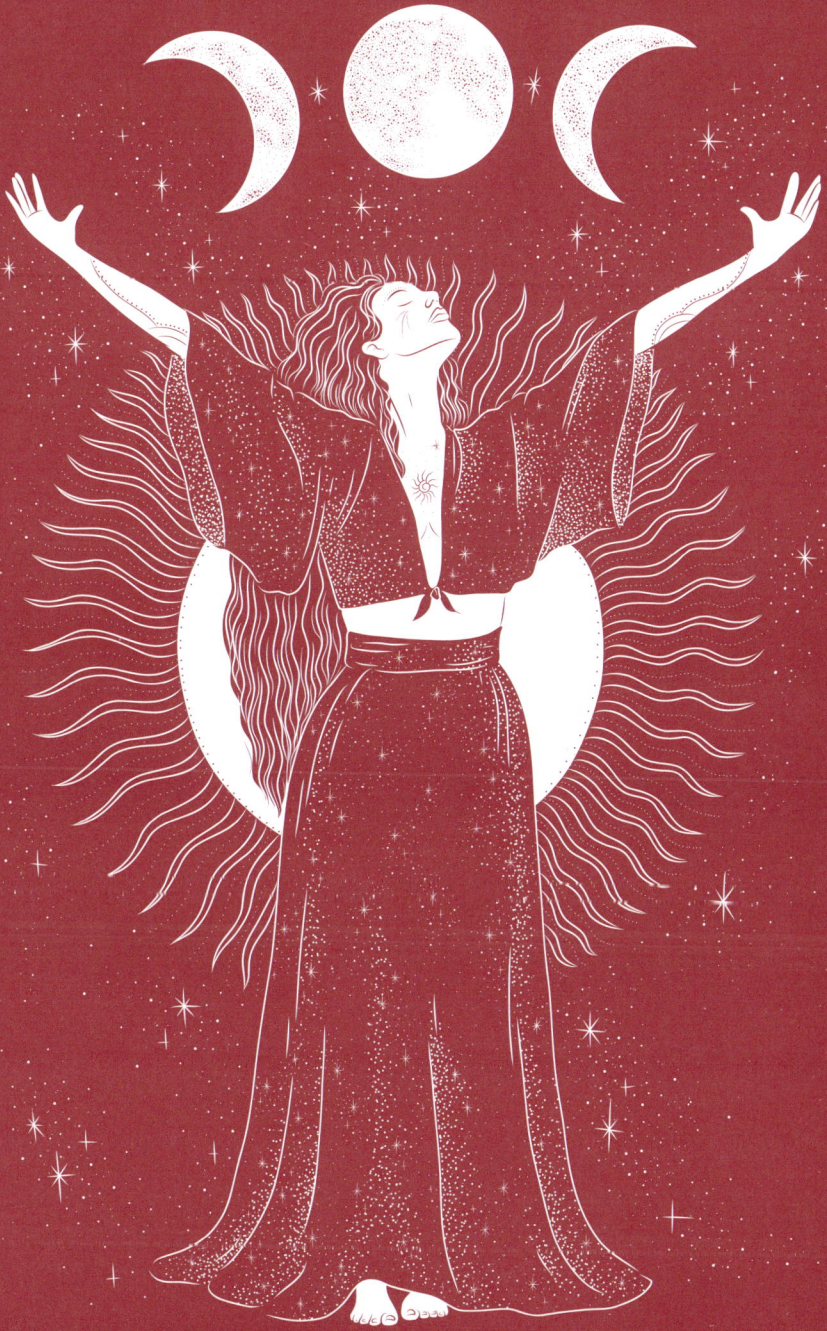

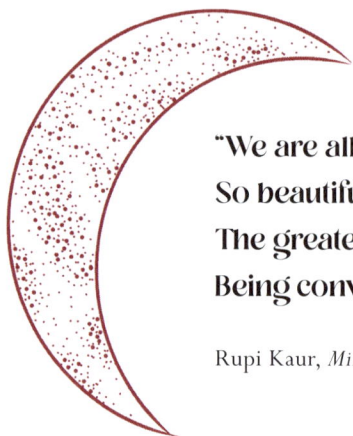

> "We are all born
> So beautiful
> The greatest tragedy is
> Being convinced we are not."

Rupi Kaur, *Milk and Honey*

Would you believe me if I told you that it wasn't always this way? That, once upon a time, our periods and our cycles weren't taboo? Instead, they were powerful and sacred.

When I talk about this in workshops, some women cock an eyebrow in disbelief. Others lean forwards and nod. They know on some level that they hold magic and wonder between their thighs.

Yet, no matter how much of this knowledge lies inside us, ready to be unearthed and unravelled, it's difficult to separate from the message that our periods are shameful. After all, we grew up with adverts for tampons and pads that showed blue liquid in place of our blood. We were told to stuff tampons up our sleeves when walking to the toilet. And many of us have only ever heard our periods spoken of in hushed whispers and euphemisms.

It takes courage to break free. For many of us, it's this message that is etched into our very bones.

And yet, if we trace our fingers back through history, there was a time where religions were Earth-based and goddesses were worshipped. In short: there was a time when women's bodies and cycles really were seen as sacred.

Sister, it's time to reclaim that narrative, and it's time to reclaim our cycles. One of the most radical, feminine things we can do is reclaim our bodies for ourselves. To refuse to see them as anything less than magical.

So, before we start to unearth some of the ancient and sacred ways, here's a thought...

What would it take for you to see your cycle in a different light?

What would it mean for you if you decided to take back your power and femininity?

And what if, right now, you made a commitment to start learning to love and cherish your body, just as you are?

Her-story

While there are many examples of history treating women badly, ancient "her-story" is very different.

Our wombs were once seen as portals to other worlds, and our blood was believed to be the life force itself. Even the word menstruation has a more spiritual etymology. It stems from the word *menses*, which has roots in the word "moon". Long ago, communities recognised how a woman's cyclical nature meant that she was forever entwined with Mother Nature and the moon.

Archaeologists have found evidence of goddess worship from around the world – in Egypt, Greece, South America, and countless other regions. In fact, some of the earliest-surviving artefacts that have been found prove that we are living in what was once a feminine world.

In Avebury, England, there's an ancient circle of stones which many believe represent the Goddess', or the Great Mother's, womb. Moving to Ancient Greece, and the sacred and ancient site of Delphi translates to mean "womb". Once upon a time in Greek her-story – long before Aristotle held that if a woman looked in a mirror when she was bleeding, it would cloud over – menstrual blood was believed to offer protection.

Meanwhile, sculptures of heavy-bellied, large-breasted Venuses (such as the Venus of Willendorf) have been found dotted around Europe, and as far away as Siberia. There are also countless carved figures, known as Sheela na gig, which feature prominent vulvas. Even now, you can still find these carvings on many ancient churches.

Speaking of vulvas (how often can you say that phrase?), throughout her-story there have been tales and myths told of women flashing their vulvas to prevent evil, or to represent their power, or to help to nurture and support life.

Once upon a time, it was even thought that women would lift their skirts to encourage crops to grow. In Greek mythology, the goddess Demeter sank into a deep depression when Persephone was abducted by Hades and taken to the Underworld. Demeter travelled the world in search of her beloved daughter, growing more and more depressed as she did so.

As she tumbled into the depths of despair, the world shrivelled. Crops perished, and the land grew parched, until Demeter met Baubo, an elderly lady. Baubo did what no one else had been able to: she made the goddess howl with laughter by lifting her skirts and flashing her vulva. This gave Demeter the strength to find her daughter and bargain with Hades so that she could be returned to Earth for six months of the year.

The power of the vulva!

Meanwhile, Inanna, the beautiful Mesopotamian goddess of love and sex, was renowned for the beauty of her anatomy. The goddess's vulva was seen as sacred (it was described in texts as a "boat of heaven", or a "lap of honey"). In an ancient Sumerian text, *Inanna, Queen of Heaven and Earth*, she was described like this: "When she leaned against the apple tree, her vulva was wondrous to behold. Rejoicing at her wondrous vulva, the young woman Inanna applauded herself."

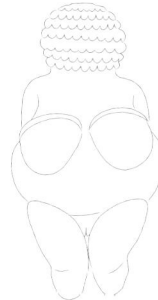

The Venus of Willendorf

For those of us who have grown up feeling as though our bodies are ugly or shameful – especially our vulvas – this description can seem astonishing. Even more so when you learn that ancient terms for our anatomy (many of them originating in the Far East) included Golden Lotus, Dragon's Pearl, Jade Gateway, and Precious Pearl.

Compare this to the poisonous words and phrases we hear hurled at women today (I refuse to list them – I'm sure you know them). If you haven't already, imagine the impact this may have had on your beautiful body as you grew up – the stress and shame this has caused you to store.

If you'd grown up hearing female bodies talked about in sacred whispers instead, how might life have been different?

Viva la vulva indeed.

What Happened?

While I love to focus on the sacredness of our cycles, it's important to understand what happened.

Sadly, we'd need an entire book to unearth and uncover all the ways in which women have had their power eroded (ultimately by men) over the years. Yet, this isn't a rant against the patriarchy, which has also done damage to countless men. It's a short history of the ways in which women have had their bodies controlled.

After all, who can forget that, in the Bible, Eve was cast as the source of sin? Her punishment was to be shunned, and to experience painful periods and labour. In the Bible's *Leviticus*, men are urged not to touch menstruating women: "Whenever a woman has her menstrual period, she will be unceremonially unclean for seven days".

With the rise of Christianity and other religions, many of the ancient Goddess and Earth-based communities died out, or were forced underground. The power of women's bodies was slowly fading.

Over the years, as Christianity became more and more popular – and with men holding all the power – texts suggested that women who were bleeding were faulty and inferior.

In *Unwell Women*, author Elinor Cleghorn tells of a book known as *Secrets of Women*, published in the 13th or 14th century. The book was written by a man and was aimed at monks and priests. However, it was used to cast menstruation as the root of a woman's sins. In it, the author wrote that our blood could corrupt or even infect.

Slowly but surely, female healers, midwives, and doctors were actively discouraged. Around the 14th century, universities banned women from studying medicine.

Over the centuries that followed, even our sacred anatomy has been laid claim to by men – our G-spots, fallopian tubes, and Kegel muscles were all named after the men who "discovered" them.

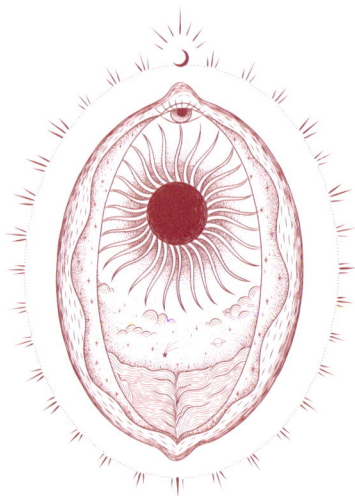

Angry Yet?

Hysteria was also used to dismiss and deride women for centuries. The term stems back to Aristotle, who first talked about the "wandering womb" (*hystera* is Greek for womb) and its myriad symptoms, which included "excessive emotion". In fact, "hysteria" was still able to be used as a catch-all way to diagnose all that could possibly be wrong with women until 1980, when it was finally removed from medical diagnostic manuals.

In the centuries that followed Aristotle, powerful women continued to be silenced and shunned. During the witch trials (most prevalent in the 17th century), women around the world were murdered for the sin of being "witches". These women were often among the wisest, most powerful women of their communities – the healers, the midwives, the medicine women. Other powerful women were encouraged to turn in their loved ones, their friends, and their sisters, to save their own lives.

The act of silencing women – of pitting them against one another – had begun.

At the same time, history was erased and rewritten. Many books were burned and destroyed during the Middle Ages, possibly causing many ancient, feminine arts (among other works) and ways of healing to be lost.

In more recent centuries, women were commonly treated for "fragile" nervous systems, using cures such as genital massages (which were given by medical providers).

The lesser-known Contagious Diseases Act was written into law in Victorian England. During this stretch of her-story, women who were believed to be sex workers (note the word "believed" here) could end up having to be forcibly examined by doctors to see if they carried any STDs. Under the Act, they could be held in "lock hospitals", imprisoned away from their families, their friends, and their loved ones.

Shockingly, even now, the echoes of this history remain. Women are still more likely to be diagnosed with mental illnesses, or have their pain described as "psychosomatic".

This is just a brief history of her-story – because, truthfully, I could write an entire encyclopedia on this subject. Yet, it's important to recognise this: in societies where a woman's power was recognised and revered, our menstrual cycles and our bodies were held as sacred.

On the flip side, in societies where a woman's power was feared, our cycles have been shrouded in shame.

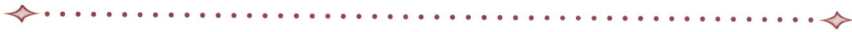

Menstrual Blood

Given all this, it's little wonder that so many of us are ashamed of our blood.

Yet, let's finish this section with celebration: far from being gross and gory, our menstrual blood is powerful. In fact, modern science is starting to play catch up – and our blood is (finally) now being studied and researched to see how it can be used to heal.

As I write this, the amazing scientist Christine Metz has found a way for our menstrual blood to be used to test more quickly for endometriosis. Other researchers are studying menstrual blood to see if it can be used to speed up wound healing, treat heart conditions, and even slow the progress of Parkinson's disease.

When you consider that period blood is known to be rich in healing stem cells, you can see why it's starting to be seen as such a precious substance, a potential elixir.

So, you see, there's magic, power, and wonder in our cycle. In the words of the author Lara Owen: your period blood is gold.

Your Body is an Altar

Now we know what "his-tory" has done to women, we need to start rewriting the narrative: and that comes with daring to see your own beautiful body as sacred, as an altar to Goddess herself.

A large part of my own personal healing journey has lain in learning to love my body. It took a lot of work – both with therapists, and with myself – so I'm not going to be flippant. If you struggle with your own body image, reading a few words by me is unlikely to change that. You likely need (and deserve) support from a professional.

Yet, your body truly is an altar.

No matter the number on the scales (I'll take this opportunity right now to say this: please stop weighing yourself), no matter how many laughter lines etch your face with their stories, and no matter how many stretch marks or threads of cellulite snake their way across your form: your body is an altar.

You are a representation of Goddess herself. You are perfect, you are beautiful, and you are whole – just as you are.

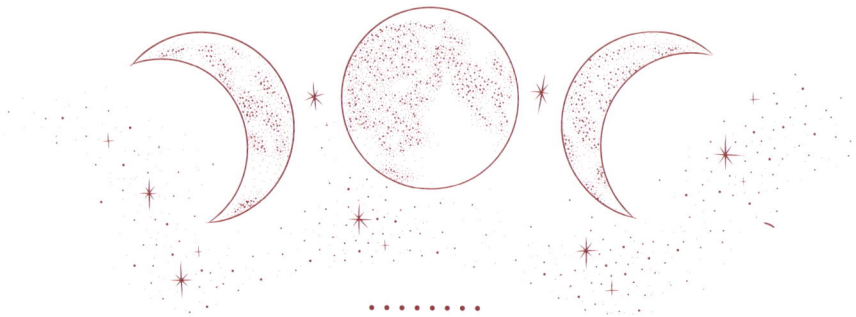

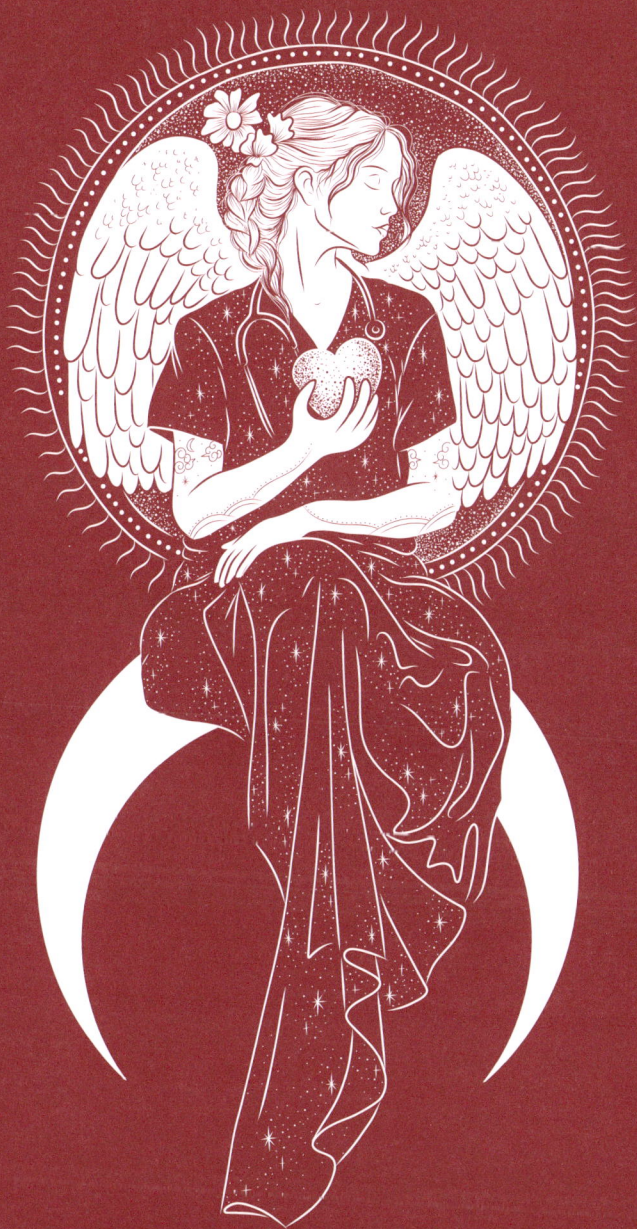

Sacred Power
Exercise

✧ • • • • • • • • • • • • • • • • • • ✧

Over the next few days, I'd like you to connect to your sacred self. If we're really going to heal our hormones, we have to dig deeper than biology alone – we have to learn to wear our feminine crowns with pride. We can start by treating our bodies with love, tenderness, and sensuality – even if we aren't quite there with our thoughts.

So, massage yourself with beautifully-fragranced oils. Run yourself a hot bath with flowers, salts, and oils – and luxuriate in it.

Wear clothes and knickers that make you feel sexy and confident, Every. Single. Day. Don't wait around for a special occasion. If you feel drawn to, don't wear knickers at all!

Look in the mirror and smile at yourself. Tell yourself how beautiful you are. Wink at your reflection. Blow yourself seductive kisses. Admire the softness of your skin, or lounge around in a silk kaftan eating juicy, seasonal fruits or dark chocolate.

Try the Vulva Gazing exercise in the Summer chapter.

Make yourself the chocolate cake in the Winter chapter, just because!

Take yourself out on a solo date – because whose company could possibly be better than your own?

Shake and wriggle your hips to your favourite songs, or twerk and writhe to a sensual play list.

Buy yourself flowers, or a new book to read.

And slowly but surely, you will come to see yourself as the sacred goddess that you are.

With this in mind, now – or whenever you feel ready to – take a moment to ask yourself:

· What things do I do to honour my body?

· How would I like to honour my body?

· What makes me feel good about myself, or what makes me feel sensual and sexy?

· What do I enjoy?

· How can I honour my body as sacred every single day?

Whatever it is, set aside time for yourself to indulge in this. Every day, for a whole week.

By the end of the week, ask yourself: did I feel any differently about myself when I was choosing to do these things? What changed or shifted? Did I feel any resistance?

If it felt good to you, if it helped you to shift into honouring yourself as sacred and divine...what's stopping you from doing this more?

Magical Facts

Finally, before we move onwards, here are some magical facts about your beautiful, female body. Try reading these and telling me you aren't a goddess embodied:

· The tissue in the vagina is the same tissue that lines the mouth. In fact, there's a huge connection between our pelvic bowl and the throat/jaw and mouth. This is one of the reasons why it's so important to sing, hum, and use your voice wherever you can.

· Our eggs are the largest cells in the human body – and the only ones visible to the human eye. When an egg is fertilised by sperm, it emits a halo of light – like a tiny, shimmering firework display. This spark occurs as zinc is released. When you look at it like this, you can see how much energy you really need to start this process.

· Our vulvas are as unique as snowflakes. Each one is different and beautiful in its own way.

· When we ovulate, both our cervical mucus and our saliva look like crystallised fern leaves when viewed through a microscope. It's a process known as "ferning".

· Like Matryoshka dolls, women begin their cellular lives as eggs, nestled safely in their grandmother's tummy. This is because the majority of eggs we carry (perhaps all eggs – more research needs to be done!) form in our ovaries when we are four-month-old foetuses, held in the wombs of our mothers.

Your Cycle is Sacred

After reading this, I hope you're able to start questioning the narrative you may have felt for most of your life.

But, above all, I hope you can start to see yourself through a new lens. A lens of love, magic, and wonder. Because, believe me, your cycle is your super power. Your cycle is sacred. And you, right in this very moment, are a divine, shimmering, and beautiful goddess.

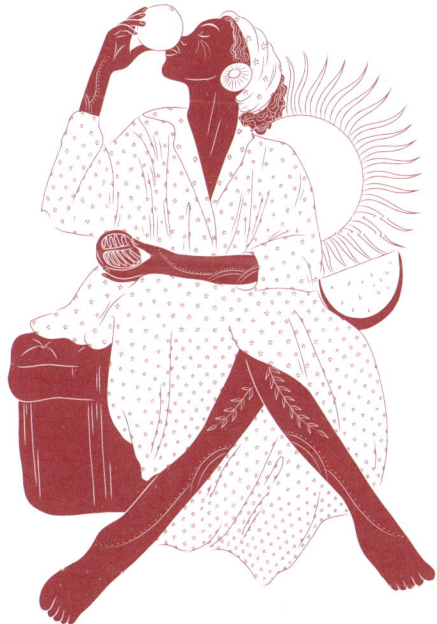

Meet your Hormones

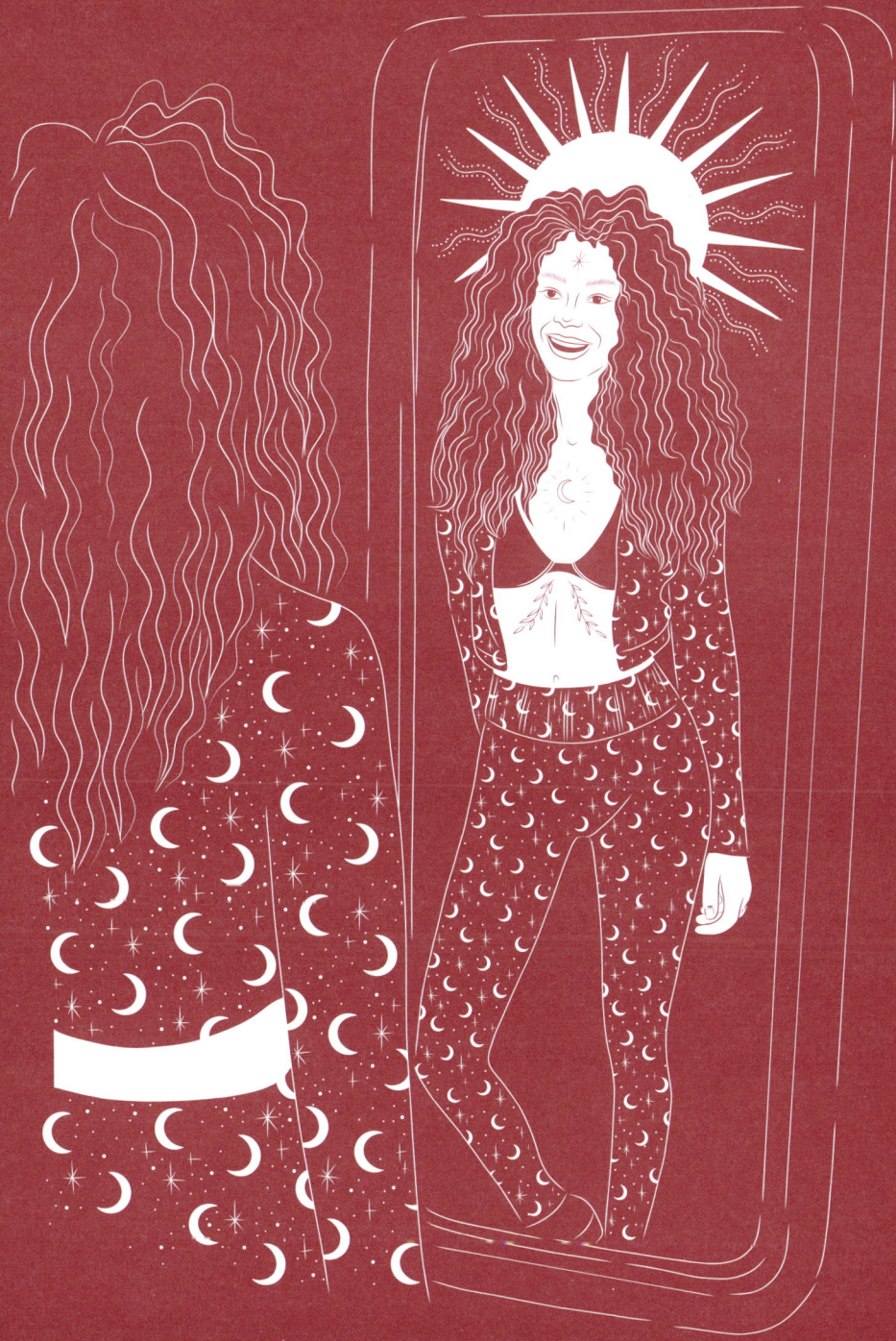

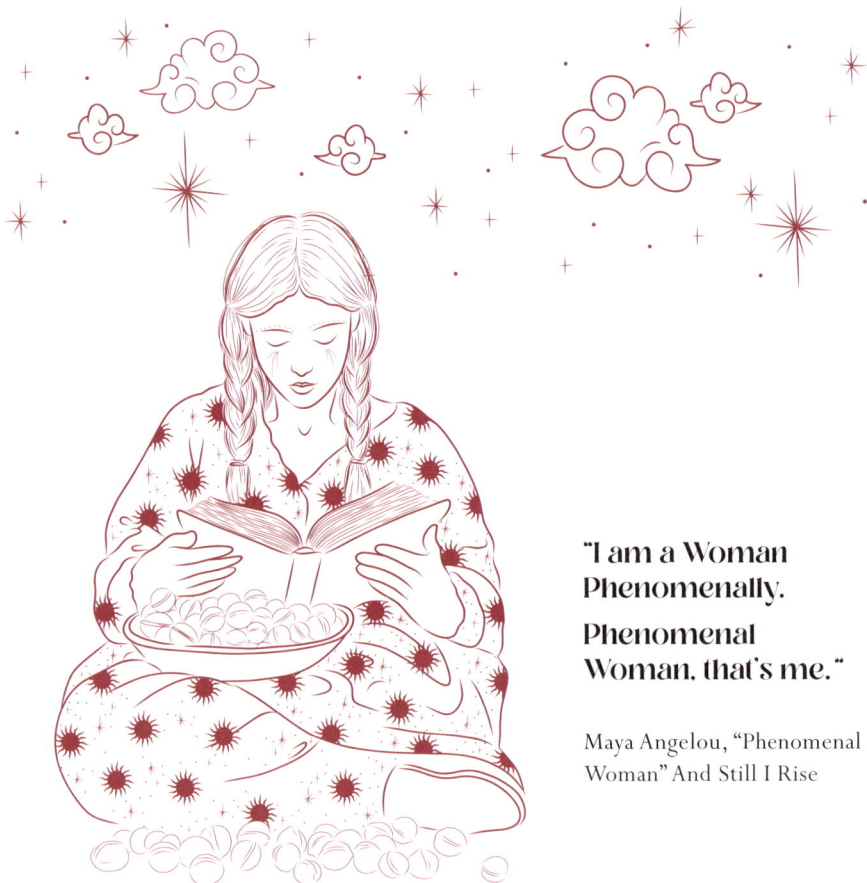

> "I am a Woman
> Phenomenally.
> Phenomenal
> Woman, that's me."

Maya Angelou, "Phenomenal
Woman" And Still I Rise

It may be a cliché, but it's a cliché because it's true: knowledge is power. And a woman empowered with knowledge about her body and her cycle – who knows she holds magic between her thighs – is an unstoppable force. By the end of this book, that empowered woman is going to be you. But before we get you there, we need to dive a little deeper and line those foundations. For some of you this section might seem a bit heavy, but bear with me – it's important, and it's going to help you to understand your body.

What Are Hormones?

Given that we are often taught so little about our bodies, we'll start with the real basics. So, what the heck are hormones anyway?

Simply put, hormones are chemical messengers. While you might associate them with your menstrual cycle, we have hormones for all kinds of things. In fact, there are more than 50 different kinds of known hormones in the body! There's a hormone for hunger (ghrelin), and a hormone which tells us when we're full (leptin). There's a hormone to help us sleep (melatonin), and there's even a hormone which helps us to love and build trust (oxytocin). In short: there's a hormone for pretty much everything.

However, for the purposes of this book, we're going to be focusing on our sex hormones. These include oestrogen, progesterone, and testosterone (yes, women need testosterone too!), which need cholesterol to form. Despite what you may or may not hold onto from the era of low-fat diets, this is why it's essential you let go of that old, ancient messaging and eat plenty of healthy fats.

Anyway, while you might loathe and curse your sex hormones, the reality is: we need them all. And, ideally, we need them to work in harmony and in symphony.

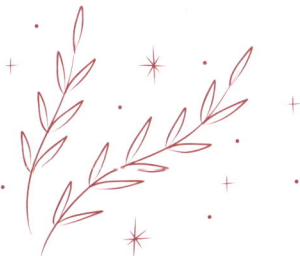

Hormone Imbalances

If your hormones feel a little wayward, then you are not alone. As we've already learned, it's thought that 80–90% of women struggle (or have struggled) with their hormones in some way or another.

From the first chapter of this book, you learned about some of the symptoms of imbalances, include bloating, migraines, heavy bleeding, painful periods, breast tenderness, and more. We'll go much deeper into the symptoms of specific hormonal imbalances in this chapter.

Yet, it's also important to point out that these symptoms can be related to other underlying issues and health concerns. And, trendy as it may be to blame our hormones for Every. Last. Thing., I can promise you that it's not always their fault. In fact, hormonal imbalances are often a symptom, rather than a root cause.

In the women I see, the root cause is often that their bodies don't feel safe – which is why the nervous system work in the Hormone 101 chapter later in this book is so important. Yet, I'd advise you to check out any persistent symptoms with your doctor before you do anything else.

What's normal anyway?

On the flip side, we don't want to be all doom and gloom. It's also important to know when we're doing something right.

While all women are different – there's no "one size fits all", and I encourage you to explore what *your* signs of health are – here are some signs that your hormones are thriving:

· You wake feeling hungry.

· You fall asleep (and stay asleep) easily.

· You have a healthy libido (although, ladies, our libido is complex – it's tied to much more than just hormone health).

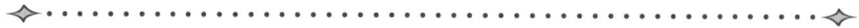

- Your period lasts for 3–7 days.
- When you have your period, your blood is bright red with little to no clottting. However, it is normal to have some dark brown or darker red blood at the start and end of your bleed.
- Your menstrual cycle is fairly regular.
- You feel energised, vibrant, and – generally – in control of things.
- You wake up feeling rested.
- You have regular bowel movements (at least once at day).
- You have warm hands and feet.
- You rarely experience bloating or any other digestive issues.
- You get excited by your loves, passions, and dreams.
- You feel in control of your emotions.
- You can maintain your body's ideal weight without extreme methods.

If you check off most of the things on this list, congratulations – you're well on the way! However, please also remember that healing isn't linear.

Sometimes, no matter how much we get to grips with our bodies, no matter how much work we do on ourselves, our hormones can slip – and we can experience all kinds of symptoms we thought we'd already addressed.

Life can happen. Traumas can happen, stressors can happen. No matter how much you follow the advice in this book, it's unlikely that you'll sail through life with completely perfect periods from this moment onwards – and that's OK.

I struggle with bumps in the road at times too! The key thing is that you'll be learning ways to support your body – even through the hardest of times.

What causes imbalances?

Truthfully, all kinds of things.

Again, it's important to get to the bottom of why you're experiencing these symptoms – you can only really treat hormonal issues once you've dug deeper and pulled up the roots.

Our hormones – just like our bodies and minds – are complex. Symptoms of hormonal imbalances can be triggered by:

- Emotional pain and traumas
- High inflammation (which can be caused by stress, poor diet, allergies, and more)
- Chronic gut imbalances
- Poor nutrition
- Mineral imbalances, such as low magnesium
- A sluggish liver
- Chronically high stress, including over-exercising
- Lack of sleep
- Endocrine disruptors (more in Hormone 101)
- Under-eating

And much more.

There are also certain conditions that can cause or worsen hormonal symptoms. For example, PMS can be magnified if you have autism or ADHD, while mood changes – along with chronic fatigue or brain fog – could indicate thyroid issues. Chronic bloating and cramping are also common in women with endometriosis or PCOS.

This is why it's so important that you speak to a doctor if you are experiencing any symptoms, especially if they're stubbornly holding on.

Infradian Rhythm

Another reason why women struggle so much with their hormones is because the world we live in beats to the rhythm of male hormones and the circadian rhythm.

The circadian rhythm is our 24-hour sleep/wake cycle. Quite simply, it tells us when to feel awake and alert, and when we need to rest and sleep.

Our "Hustle Culture" (think your typical nine-to-five office job) runs to this rhythm – we set our alarms and wake when cortisol levels should be rising (cortisol helps to wake us up and should peak at roughly 7–8am). And then we get to work and set about rushing, doing, and pushing.

We come home, wind down, and scramble into bed – exhausted – when cortisol has (in theory) dropped, and the sleep hormone melatonin starts to take over.

The next day, we start the cycle again: rinse and repeat, ad infinitum, without ever stopping to breathe, to rest, or to adjust and change, and to slow down.

The problem?

This isn't what our beautiful female hormones need.

While women have a circadian rhythm too – which I'll stress again, is also important for our health and our hormones (more about this in the Hormone 101 chapter) – we are also cyclical beings. But we are vastly different to men, and modelling our health and our daily schedules on a man's inner body clock can do us more harm than good. Women need more sleep, for example, and we also need more body fat to thrive. On top of this, we have what's known as an "infradian rhythm".

Infradian rhythms differ in length from woman-to-woman, but they're typically around 28 days long. In essence, it's the length of your entire menstrual cycle – running from day one of your bleed, right up until your next period.

While it may sound complicated and scientific, it doesn't need to be. All you really need to know is that your infradian rhythm circles around your hormones. Just like the moon, just like the seasons, just like the tides, women ebb and flow through the month. We shift and change as our hormones shift and change.

As you'll come to learn, this means that our needs also shift and change. We aren't meant to constantly bash through to-do lists, pump out endless work and reams of ideas.

So: women aren't "mini men". We aren't meant to live the same day-to-day routine, or even week-to-week, and we shouldn't be expected to push through and fight harder when we are feeling tired and depleted.

The longer we live in this high-speed, hectic, masculine world, the more chaos can start to stir within our beautiful female bodies.

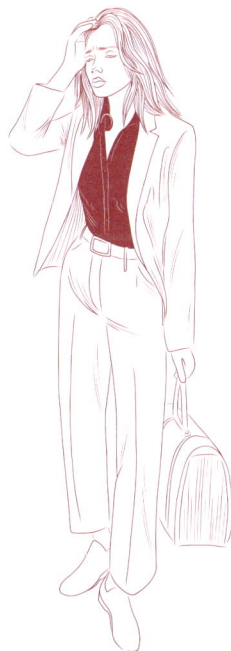

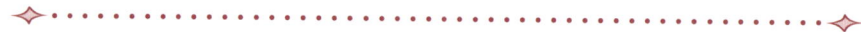

A Word on Emotions

Again, a reminder that, while your hormones are crucial for so much in the body, our emotions aren't separate entities.

It's simple to read this chapter and think, "darn my high cortisol" – and yet, our symptoms often go much deeper than this.

Hormonal imbalances don't always have physical roots. In fact, they often have emotional roots. If you are struggling, please consider the impact that your thoughts, relationships, finances, trauma, sex life, home life, and even career may be having on your health.

Finally, before we meet your hormones, please remember that change takes time – and results rarely happen overnight. In fact, our eggs take 90 days to mature, so what you do today can impact your cycle health in three months – something to bear in mind if you're struggling!

Introducing Your Hormones

In all honesty, we could spend an entire book learning about each and every single one of your hormones.

However, we don't really need to do that. For now, we'll focus on the main players of your cycle, although I encourage you to read further if you're curious.

As we dive deeper, you may notice that many of the symptoms of hormonal imbalances bleed into one another. This is partly because our hormones are meant to work in harmony with one another – when one is out of synch, the others will also shift and change.

For instance, it's very common to experience signs of oestrogen dominance at the same time as low progesterone. Since cortisol also has a big say in our menstrual cycle, you may experience many symptoms of high cortisol, as well as low progesterone, or oestrogen dominance.

It's no wonder we can find things so tricky...

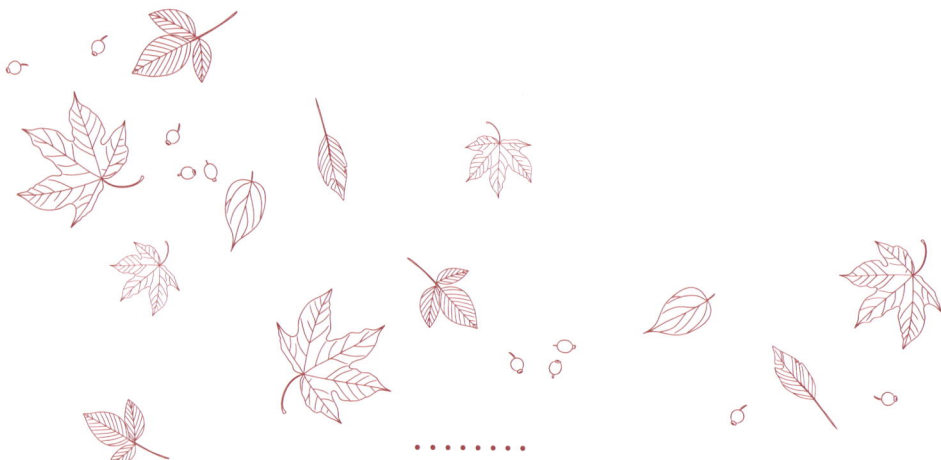

Oestrogen

This is the hormone that most of us know, love – and also love to hate.

I see oestrogen as the sassiest member of the "Sex Hormone Family" – she likes to act the star, and she demands all the attention. However, as with most things in life: you can have too much of a good thing.

A woman's oestrogen is mostly made in the ovaries (although your adrenals and even fat cells can play a part), but can also be produced by the placenta during pregnancy. There are also different kinds of oestrogen... but let's not complicate things too much.

Oestrogen ebbs and flows throughout our cycle, peaking just before ovulation. It then rises a second time (but less sharply) in our luteal phase, about a week before we start our periods. Oestrogen level are at their lowest point when we start our bleed, which is why many women find that this is when they feel most tired, less sociable, and easily depleted.

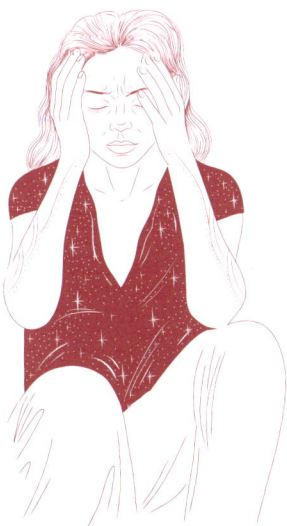

Oestrogen is necessary for ovulation, and it helps to thicken the uterine lining (aka the endometrium) ready for potential fertilisation. However, it's also crucial for many other things: libido, confidence, sexual pleasure and arousal, as well as heart health, memory, bone health, and skin health. This is why our menstrual cycles are crucial – even if we don't want to get pregnant!

So, we need oestrogen – she may be sassy, but she's crucial for our health, and we can't be without her.

When oestrogen becomes a problem...

Unfortunately, oestrogen likes to dominate – and this is when things can spiral out of control.

For this reason, oestrogen dominance is one of the most common hormonal imbalances I see. However, symptoms of this don't necessarily mean soaring levels of oestrogen. In fact, it's possible to experience symptoms of oestrogen dominance, even when you're low in the hormone. Confusingly, it's all about balance – and, in particular, it's all about the balance between oestrogen and progesterone.

When levels of oestrogen are high in relation to progesterone, this is when you can experience symptoms of PMS, as well as fibroids, fibrocystic breasts, and more.

So, how do we get there? Well, imbalanced oestrogen can be caused and triggered by many things, such as poor liver or gut health, chemical disruptors found in our environment, chronic stress, inflammation, poor diet, obesity, and more. It's also common for oestrogen to swing wildly when we are perimenopausal.

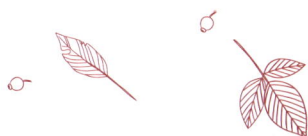

Often, hormonal imbalances are caused by more than one, or even all, of the aforementioned.

Signs you may be struggling with oestrogen dominance include:

- Heavy periods (often with clots)
- Migraines and headaches
- PMS
- Water retention
- Breast tenderness
- Mood swings
- Painful periods
- Weight gain

Low oestrogen

On the flip side, low oestrogen is also a common issue. You can have too much of a good thing – and you can also have not enough at all.

One of the most common causes of low oestrogen is perimenopause. However, it can also point to issues such as not eating enough, excessive exercise, low body weight, or signal that your body is extremely stressed. If you are experiencing irregular or missing periods, please go and see a doctor to get checked out – there are some underlying conditions (such as Premature Ovarian Insufficiency) that can trigger these symptoms.

Worried you may be experiencing low oestrogen? Here are a few signs and symptoms indicating you may be in the thick of it:

- Fatigue
- Anxiety and/or low mood
- Weight gain
- Memory loss
- Low bone density
- Night sweats and hot flashes
- Vaginal dryness and painful sex
- Low libido
- Irregular or light periods
- Brain fog

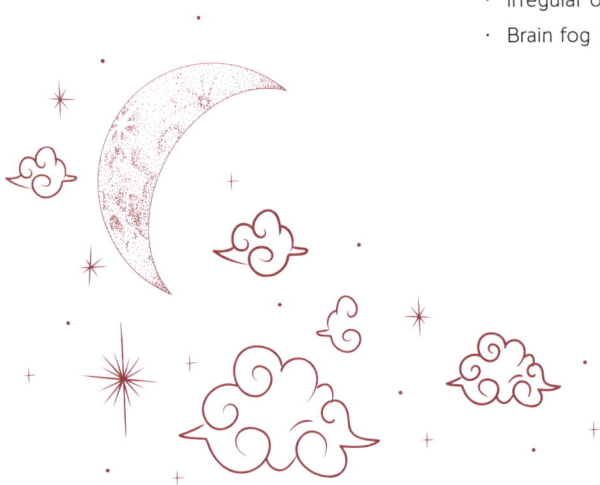

Progesterone

Like all your hormones, progesterone is a crucial player. Think of it as a backing vocalist: oestrogen may take the spotlight, but we need progesterone to have a happy, healthy, and – most importantly – calm cycle. We also need progesterone if we want to be able to get pregnant.

Progesterone is mostly secreted when the corpus luteum (the once-follicle which housed your egg) becomes a temporary endocrine gland, whose job it is to pump out the hormone. While this sounds pretty scientific, all you really need to know is this: unless we're ovulating, our bodies likely aren't benefitting from enough progesterone.

In an ideal world, our progesterone levels start to pick up the pace around ovulation. They then climb more sharply and steeply, before peaking around one week before our period.

This is progesterone working its magic, helping to maintain your uterine lining ready for potential pregnancy. However, if fertilisation doesn't take place and we don't fall pregnant, levels begin to drop, and our uterine lining will then shed (what you know as your period).

You may now be thinking: I don't want a baby. Do I still need progesterone?

Well, yes, progesterone is the calming hormone – and this is why we can all start to feel irritable, snappy, and grumpy if our bodies aren't getting enough.

Progesterone provides much-needed balance to the sass of oestrogen, and is also needed for mood. In particular, it supports the production of the neurotransmitter GABA (gamma-aminobutyric acid), which helps to keep us calm and less anxious. Progesterone is also crucial for sleep, skin, and much more.

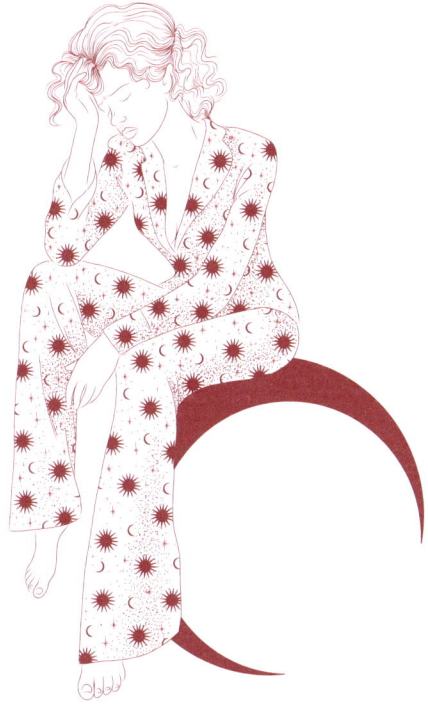

Now you know more about progesterone, it might start to make sense as to why some women experience mood changes or PMS when levels start to fall before our periods. This can be especially difficult if progesterone levels are already low, if oestrogen is too high (remember, it's all about balance!), or if your happy hormones – such as dopamine or serotonin – are low.

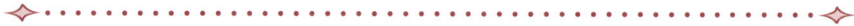

Signs of low progesterone

So, how can you tell if you're low in progesterone? Chances are you'll have experienced one of these symptoms during your cycling years – most women I work with aren't producing enough progesterone. We'll explore why in a minute, but first let's look at the symptoms:

· Infertility or frequent miscarriages

· Irritability or anxiety

· Prolonged spotting before your period

· Headaches before your period

· PMS

· Mood swings

· Poor sleep, especially before your period

· Chronic bloating, especially pre-menstrually

Causes of low progesterone

One of the main causes of low progesterone? High stress. Again, you'll be relieved to know that I won't get too scientific, but progesterone and cortisol have an intimate relationship. If we have chronically high stress levels, our bodies will channel all their efforts into creating cortisol – and progesterone gets neglected.

In other words, your body prioritises dealing with stressful situations above all else – it doesn't care about your long-term health, or whether or not you want to have a baby. It just wants to get you to safety, and it wants to get you to safety *now*.

So, if you're frazzled and stressed every day, you likely won't be making enough progesterone.

What else may be causing issues with progesterone? Anovulatory cycles, which is the fancy medical term for saying you've not ovulated, or high levels of prolactin (a hormone which is responsible for lactation when we've had a baby, but may also contribute to our stress response and more) can play a part.

Low progesterone levels are also common as we age (levels start to decline in our thirties), particularly when we are in the midst of perimenopause – it's typically the first hormone to decline. It can also occur due to an underactive thyroid, nutrient deficiencies, PCOS, and more.

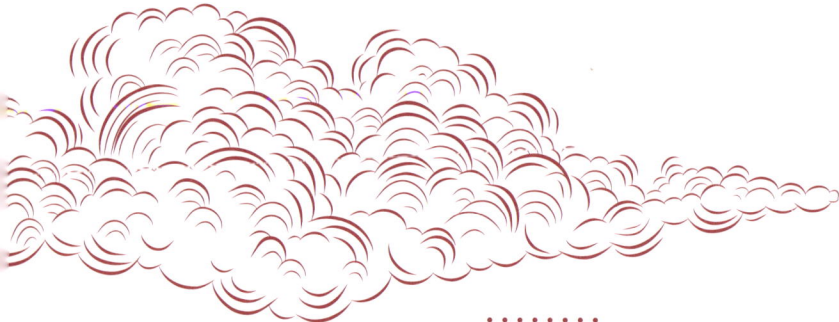

Cortisol

Moving onto a more infamous hormone, you might already know cortisol as "The Baddie", or "The Stress Hormone". As such, it often gets a toxic rep – but it's not actually all bad! Cortisol is necessary and it's also key in enabling us to focus and wake up, and to respond to life-saving situations.

The problem comes when cortisol is chronically high. Unfortunately, modern-day life is stressful for many of us – and our cortisol is often haywire as a result. As you now know, chronically high cortisol can lower progesterone. It can also impact sleep and ovulation, furthermore it can affect the thyroid, impact insulin and blood sugar levels, and obliterate our libido.

It doesn't just have to be emotional stress, either! High cortisol can be triggered by poor diet and inflammation, chronic illness, under-eating, over-exercising, food intolerances, constant exposure to hot or cold temperatures, and much more.

Signs of high cortisol include:

· Insulin resistance

· Poor sleep

· Irritability or anger

· Painful periods or PMS

· Stubborn weight gain – especially around the stomach

· Acne

· Bloating or digestive issues

· Fatigue

· Headaches

Some women will also experience low cortisol – which isn't as good as it sounds! Remember, we want our hormones to be like Goldilocks' porridge: not too much, not too little, but just right.

Low cortisol can be triggered by ongoing stress, but it can also be caused by a condition called Addison's disease, amongst other things.

Signs include:

· Extreme fatigue

· Feeling tired when you wake in the morning

· Mood swings and irritability

· Depression

· Brain fog

· Dizziness when standing

· Weight loss

· Muscle weakness

· Poor stress tolerance

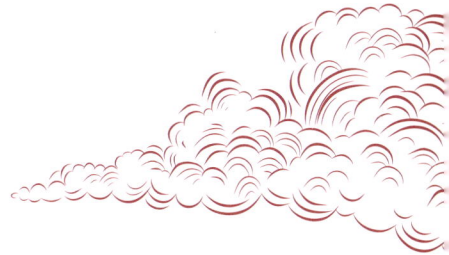

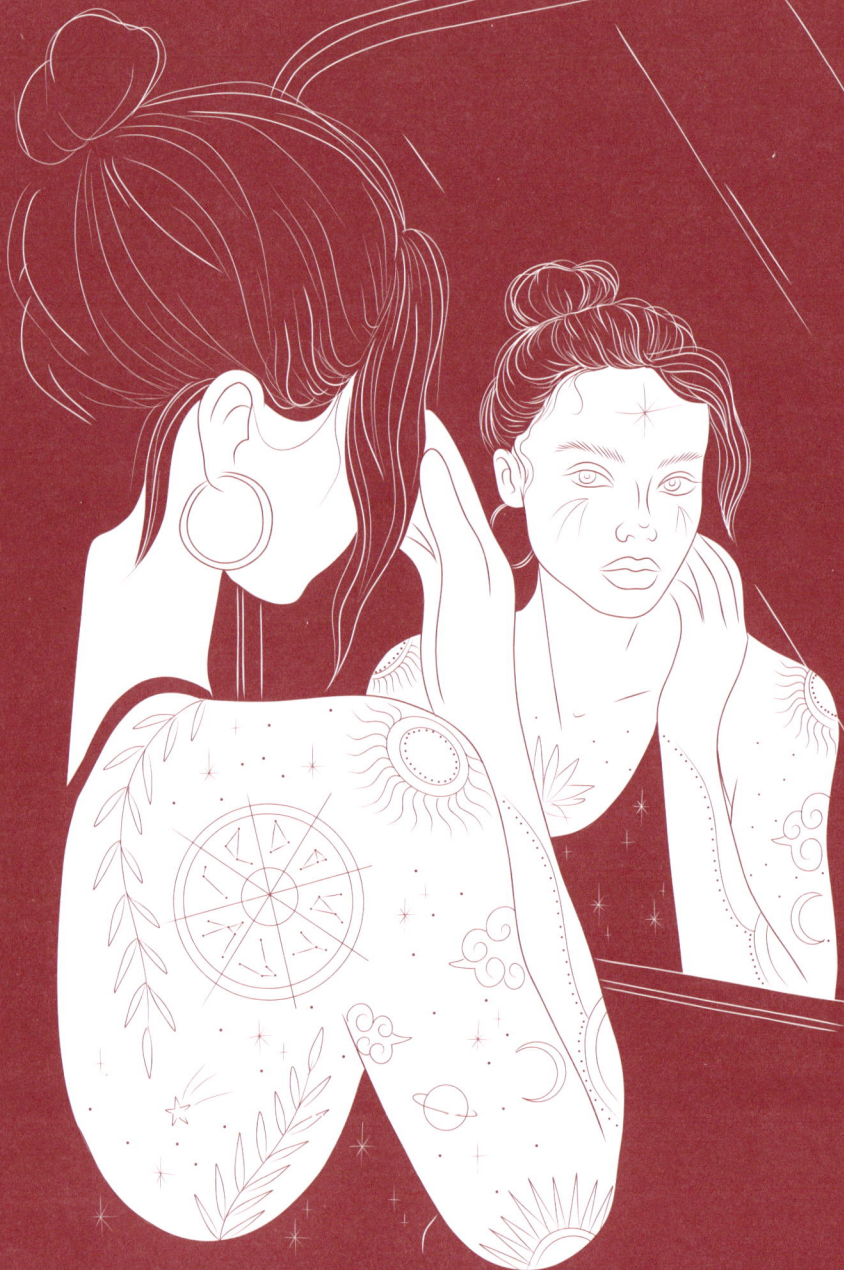

Testosterone

Just as oestrogen is more widely-associated with women, so testosterone tends to be grouped with men. However, it's also an important sex hormone in the female cycle (although in lower levels) and is made in the ovaries and adrenal glands. Testosterone is an androgen and plays a crucial part in our mood and confidence levels, as well as our memory, muscle-building capabilities, and our ability to be assertive and lay down healthy boundaries. It, too, plays a big part in ovulation. Testosterone climbs around ovulation, helping to boost sex drive and get us "in the mood".

What triggers imbalances in testosterone? High insulin levels are a major player, as are low levels of SHBG (sex hormone binding globulin), which helps to bind up the testosterone we don't need. Other issues can be caused by PCOS, an underactive thyroid, poor diets, stressors, perimenopause, trauma, and birth control.

Symptoms of high testosterone include:

· Oily skin
· Excess hair on the face and body – known as hirsutism
· Acne
· Low libido
· Thinning hair
· Deeper voice

Low testosterone symptoms include:

· Low libido
· Lack of energy
· Irregular cycle
· Depression
· Anxiety
· Thinning hair
· Loss of strength
· Brain fog

These Hormones Matter Too!

Other hormones that play a crucial role in our menstrual cycle and our hormone health include follicle stimulating hormone (FSH), luteinising hormone (LH), insulin, and thyroid hormones. If you feel curious, I'd encourage you to explore them some more!

DUTCH hormone test

Still not sure what's going on? Don't worry – things can get quite confusing, especially if multiple hormones are haywire.

If you're feeling unsure, please book in with your doctor or with a trained professional who can advise you on next steps. If you can afford it, I'd also advise you get a DUTCH test (Dried Urine Test for Comprehensive Hormones). This, as the name suggests, involves your urine being dried and tested for levels of hormones. The results can offer a really clear picture of what's going on with your cycle, which makes it easier to address and treat any issues.

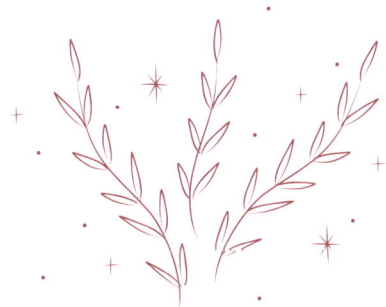

Visualisation
Exercise

Finally, before we move on, I want you to start to believe that it's possible to live your healthiest, happiest life.

After all, science now knows that our thoughts slowly turn to belief, before they seep into our cells and become our biology. In other words: your thoughts hold power.

Each day for the next few weeks or months, I'd like you to set aside five minutes to visualise a future where you are living the life of your dreams (whatever that means for you).

I'd like you to:

· Picture yourself with healthy, happy hormones.

· Picture yourself living a life where you're in tune with your body.

· Picture a version of you which is open to slowing down and resting.

· Picture a life where you fall in love with yourself, with every inch of your body – and with your period, too.

It's possible, I promise. But I want you to start believing it as much as I believe in you.

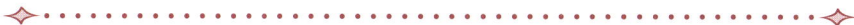

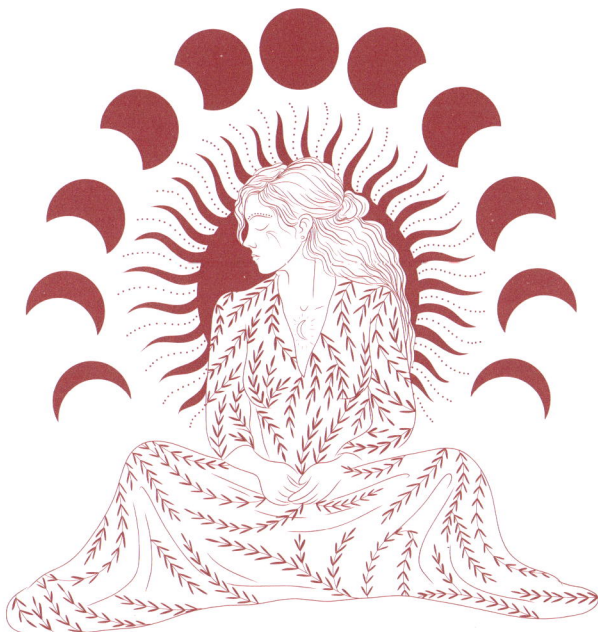

A Final Word...

Made it through this chapter? Congratulations! This is the most scientific it's going to get. It might seem like a lot to digest, but I truly believe that change can only happen if we are given this knowledge.

Now you understand your hormones, you won't be so easily fobbed off. You won't be easily ushered away, dismissed with a mere prescription for the pill, or told that all is OK simply because your blood tests are "normal". (Important point: if you feel rubbish, you deserve to be supported.)

If you're struggling with symptoms of these hormonal imbalances, I hope that things don't feel too bleak. Believe me, we're going to look at countless ways you can support your body.

Think you're ready to explore further?

Let's settle down and discover some simple ways to start bringing your hormones back into balance and alignment.

Cyclical Living

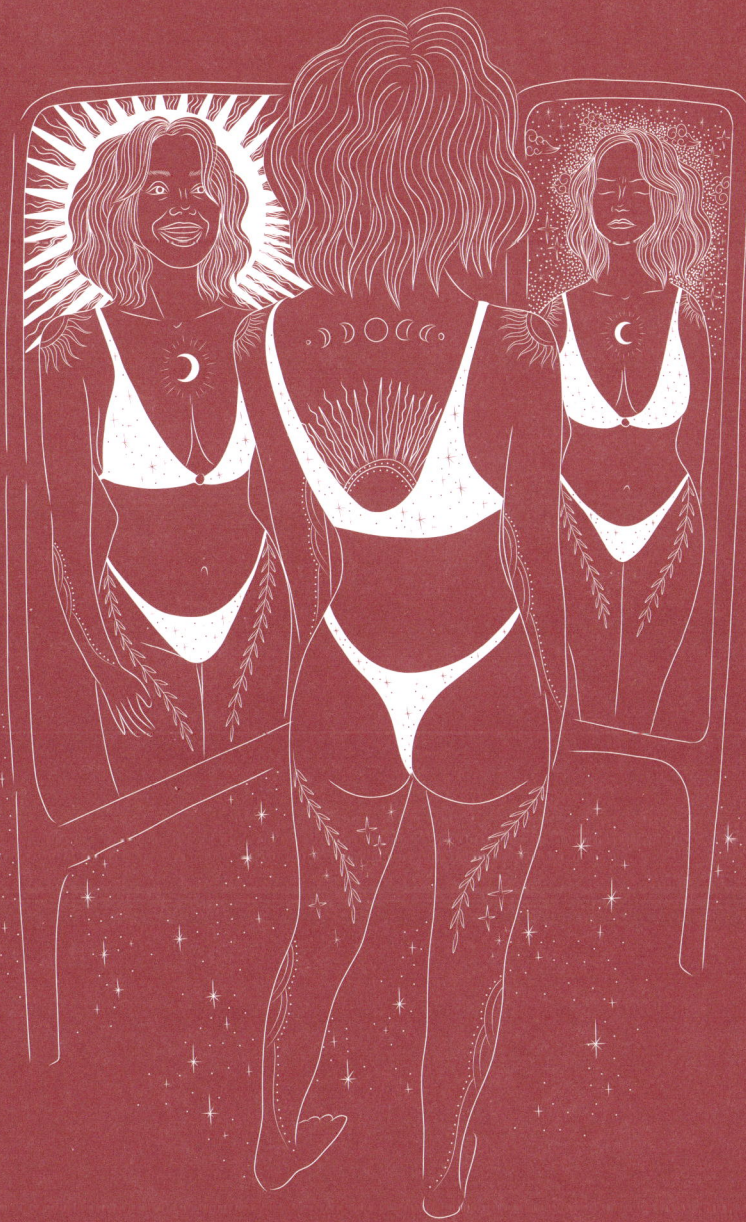

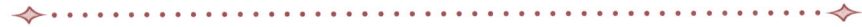

Cyclical living changed my life

It's what freed me from feeling shackled by my hormones to feeling empowered, enlightened, and free. It sounds dramatic to say it, but cyclical living is what led me to falling in love with my period – and head-over-heels in love with being a woman. No matter your hormone story, no matter where you are in your life right now, I promise that it's possible for you, too.

But, for those of you who don't know it yet: what is cyclical living?

As you hopefully now know, our hormone levels aren't the same throughout the month. They ebb and flow, shift and change. There are times where our hormones are riding high on the crest of a wave, and there are others where they plunge to the depths. In other words, we spend our cycling years spiralling.

This flow means that there are times of the month where we'll be feeling energised and vibrant, bursting with creativity and life. We'll feel sociable and magnetic, sexy, and desirable. We'll pull on our sexiest clothes, walk with heads held high, and a wiggle in our step.

Yet, there are times of the month where this flips. Where our energy pulls inwards, and we feel more easily fatigued, tired, and drained. We'll feel an urge to retreat and withdraw, and we may want to spend less time surrounded by others. We may also feel increasingly irritable, or less willing to play the role of people pleaser, as we speak our minds.

Cyclical living takes into account these waves. It helps us to live in harmony with our hormones, rather than fighting against them.

"The psyches and souls of women also have their own cycles and seasons of doing and solitude, running and staying, being involved and being removed, questing and resting, creating and incubating, being of the world and returning to the soul-place."

Clarissa Pinkola Estés,
Women Who Run with the Wolves

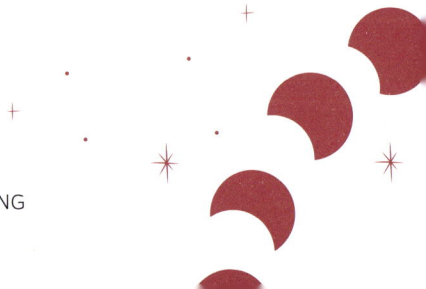

Your Phases

We'll dive into each of these phases in more detail in the following chapters, but cyclical living assumes we have four phases in our cycle. These are: winter (or your period), spring (your follicular phase), summer (ovulation), and autumn (aka your luteal phase).

Each of these phases mean we have different needs – yet they also come with their own super powers. There are no hard and fast rules, either. Rather, see it as encouragement to start listening to your body, to start understanding what you need – and to do what lights you up.

When we lean into these natural rhythms, we start to unlock the inner magic and beauty of our cycles. We stop feeling burned out and depleted. Rather than fighting against our body's natural energy levels and moods, we live in synch. We become more at peace.

By embracing cyclical living, many women – me included – effortlessly ease PMS, period pain, hormonal imbalances, or even say goodbye to them for ever.

So, you see, there's power in your hormones. There's power in your body.

No matter where you are now, no matter what you're experiencing, I promise you that the power and magic lies within you. We just need to find it – and that's what the next section will help you to do.

Cycle Tracking

If you currently don't know your cycle, or if your cycle is irregular, you might like to log your own symptoms using a journal or your phone. Each day, check in with yourself and your body and ask: what has my energy been like today? What have my physical symptoms been? Where's my sex drive at?

This will help you to get intimate with, and to understand, your own unique, beautiful body.

What if you're not bleeding or if your cycle is unpredictable?

Some women – for myriad reasons – don't bleed, while for others, cycles are unpredictable. If this is you, cyclical living is still possible. You can either tune into your own energetic needs, or you can base your cycle around the phases of the moon.

You could:

· Take the dark moon (the last vestige of the waning moon at the end of the lunar cycle) as the beginning of your cycle, or your period/winter phase.

· See the waxing moon as your follicular phase, or spring.

· Honour the full moon as ovulation, or summer.

· And lean into your luteal phase as autumn.

What if...?

Before we go any further, I'd like to take a moment to ask you to trust in yourself, and to trust in your own body.

I often tell the women I work with this: no one will ever know or understand your body better than you do. If you don't resonate with what follows, or if you feel slightly different in the phases, please trust in that.

Above all else, always be you.

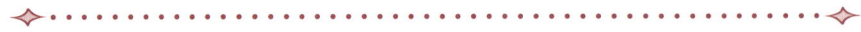

Your Hormone Cycle

The chart below shows how your hormones ebb and flow through your cycle. As you can see, when you're on your period, all hormone levels are fairly low. Oestrogen and testosterone then start to rise before peaking around ovulation. Progesterone takes over the baton as the star hormone in the second part of your cycle, before dropping right before you bleed. The second chart shows our cyclical nature – just like Mother Nature's seasons, death and rebirth are part of our everyday lives. We spiral alongside our hormones, before starting the process again.

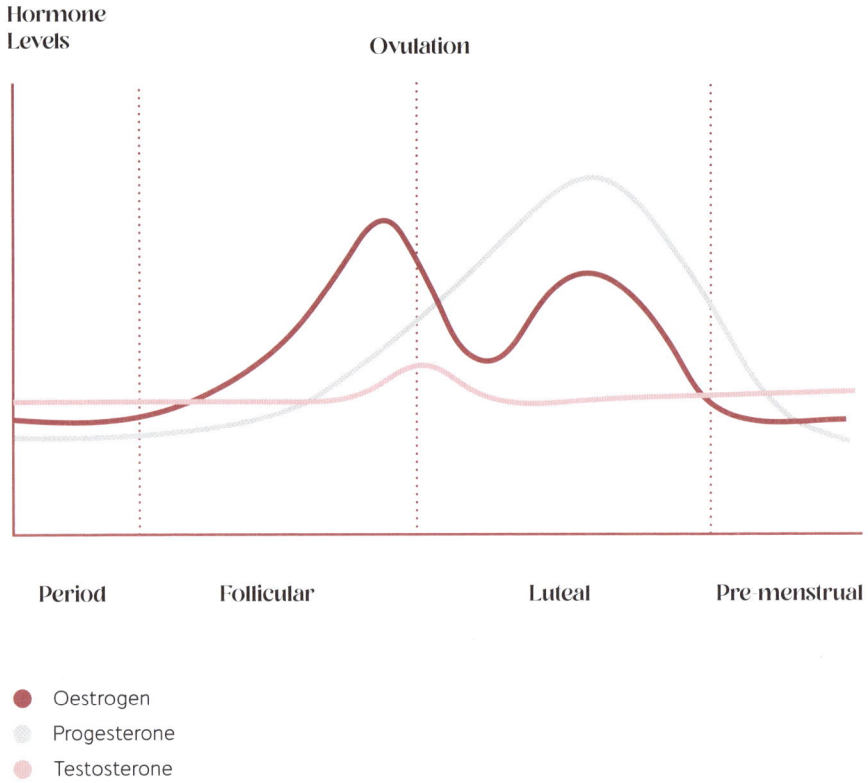

Hormone
Levels

Ovulation

Period   Follicular   Luteal   Pre-menstrual

● Oestrogen
● Progesterone
● Testosterone

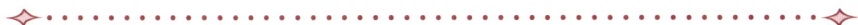

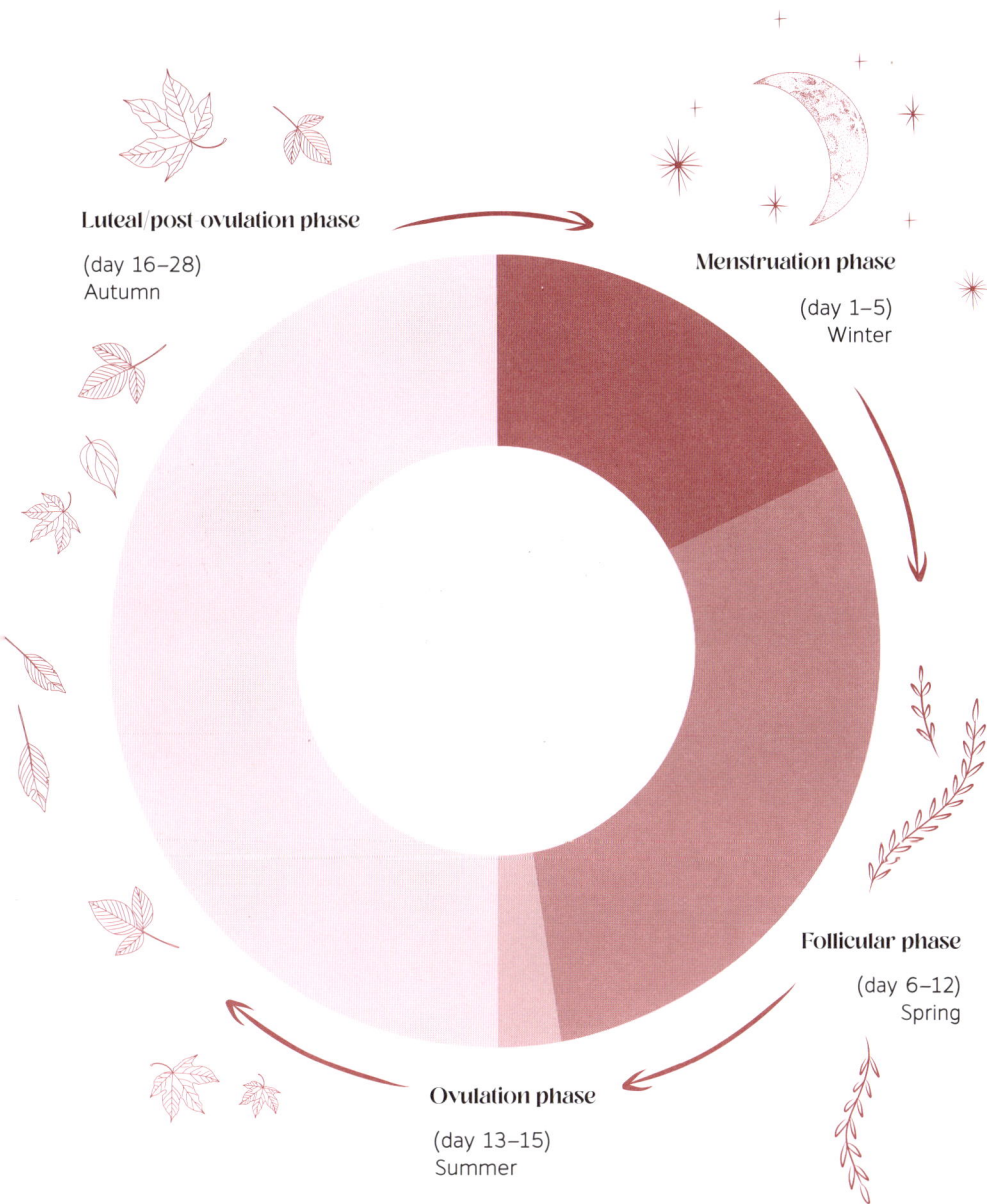

Luteal/post ovulation phase

(day 16–28)
Autumn

Menstruation phase

(day 1–5)
Winter

Follicular phase

(day 6–12)
Spring

Ovulation phase

(day 13–15)
Summer

Winter

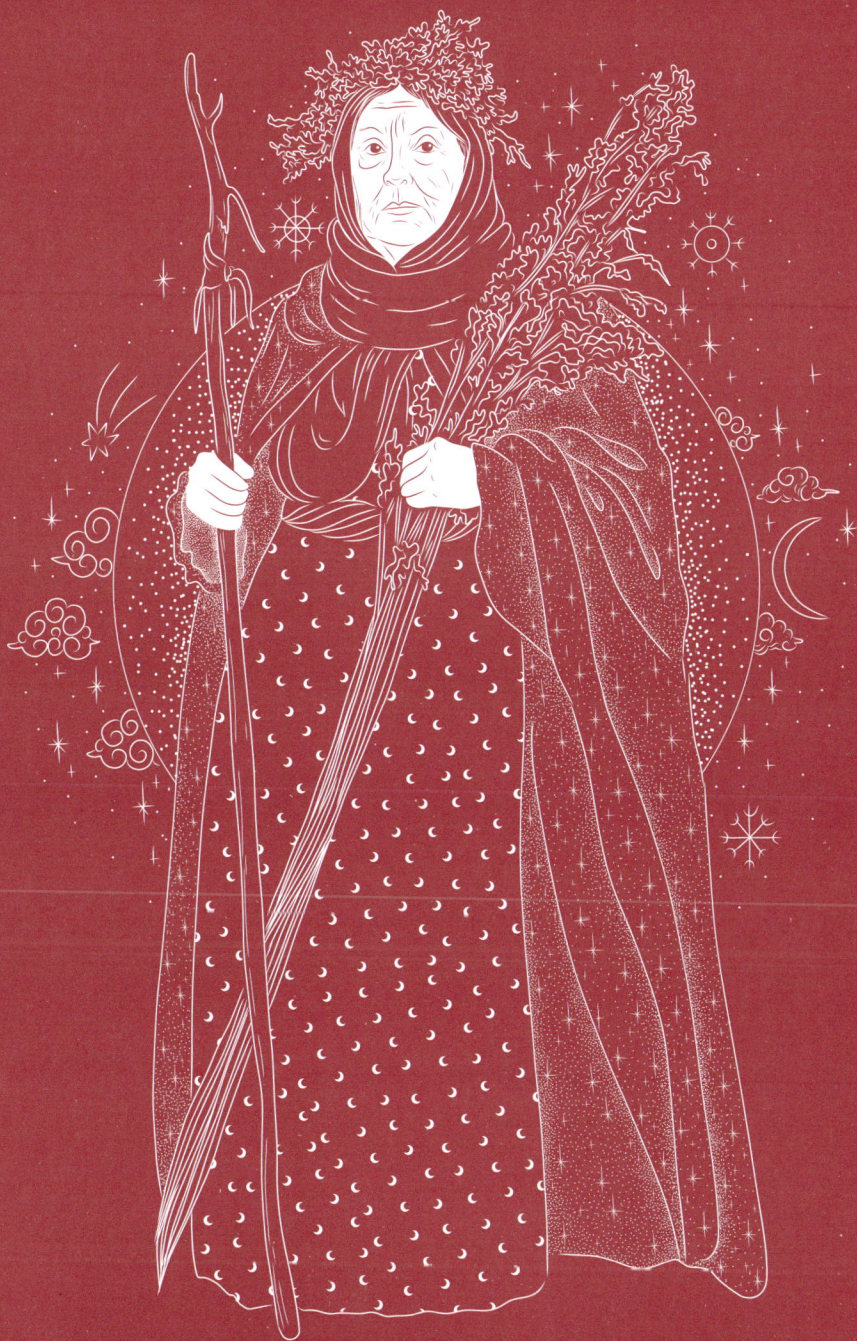

Your Period, aka Winter

Days 1–5 (approx)
of your cycle

Archetype:
Crone

Moon phase:
New moon

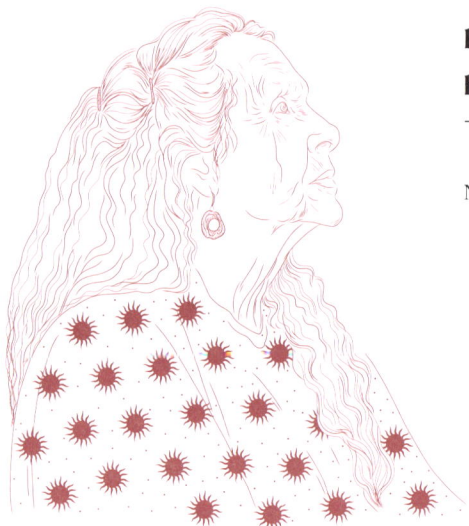

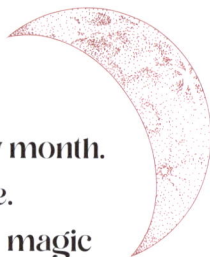

New beginnings start with an end. And so, the first day of your period welcomes in the spiral of a new cycle. Winter is ushered in when the first true blush of red blooms between our legs. For many of us, this spells the beginning of pain, cramping, and bone-aching fatigue. For others, our periods are an inconvenience – something to suffer and struggle through – and we feel giddy and gleeful when it's over. And yet, I ask you to read on with an open mind. Our "Moon Time" doesn't have to be this way. In fact, it shouldn't be this way.

"i bleed every month.
but do not die.
how am i not magic
– the lie."

Nayyirah Waheed, *Salt*

Our period is when we can command all our powers, when magic is at our fingertips, and when we can spiral, transmute, and transform.

In short: our periods are where we can step into the woman we want to be. Where we can drape ourselves in cloaks of wisdom and power, and heal wounds, breathe love into our Inner Child, and let go of limiting beliefs. Ancient communities understood this. They knew that a bleeding woman welcomed in deep wisdom and intuition. It was also understood that our periods were a time where we could start afresh, paving the way for a new chapter and new beginnings.

Our periods can be a time of great wonder, possibility and potential magic. Yet, if you struggle with period pain or suffer with conditions such as endometriosis, it's difficult to see your periods in this light. In fact, it may feel impossible.

However, while I want to acknowledge this (it's absolutely OK if you hate your bleed), please remember that you shouldn't suffer with your cycle. Period cramps, pain, heavy bleeding, and any form of suffering are not normal. If you are experiencing these things, you deserve support, and I hope that the coming pages help things to ease.

To begin with, as we delve into the first of our seasons, I ask you to simply dream.

· What if you could live your life with pain-free periods?

· What if you were able to see your periods in a different light?

· What if you were able to use your period to refill an empty cup?

Wherever you are, change is possible – even if just by one per cent. The messages I receive from women on a daily basis show this. Goddess, you really can learn to love your periods – and that's exactly what we're going to start to do.

Let's sit down together, and discover how we can harness this most primal of seasons.

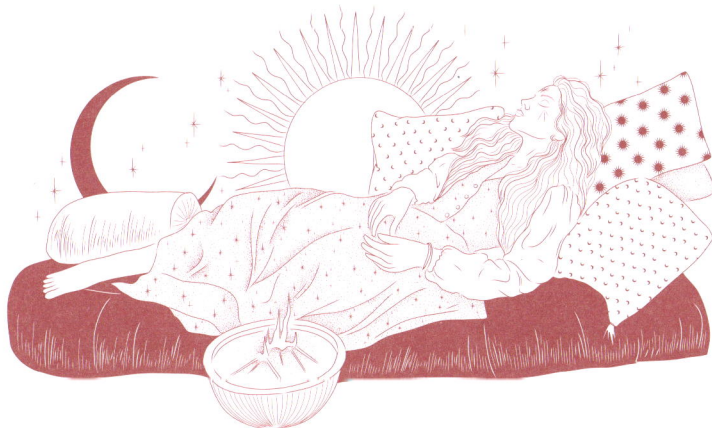

What's Happening Physically?

As you've come to read, your hormones aren't the same throughout the month – they dip and peak, trough, and then rise again. When we start our periods, our sex hormones – oestrogen, testosterone and progesterone – are at their lowest point. At the same time, prostaglandins rise so that our bodies can start shedding the uterine lining (aka the endometrium). This is what you see as blood, and this is what our period is.

For many, bleeding can bring instant relief as they lose symptoms such as breast tenderness, irritability, or anxiety. However, for others, our period is the most difficult time of the month. Symptoms you experience may include some or all of the following.

Fatigue

If you've ever felt completely wiped out, fatigued and more than a little bit "blah" on your period, this is normal! As our hormones drop to their lowest points, it's common to feel more tired than usual. Sadly, the only remedy for this is to stop fighting it! Lean into that fatigue and embrace your body's plea to slow down and rest. In fact, I have worked with many women whose period pain melts away when they slow down.

Sounds simple, but in reality this can be difficult – especially if you have kids or a full-time job.

However, consider what you can say no to. What can you put off until you enter your spring phase? And how can you refill your cup – if only by one or ten per cent?

This one shift – asking my body what it needs, and actually gifting it to myself – allowed me to fall in love with my period. If I can, I now try to take a few days off work. If this isn't possible, I immerse myself in hot salt baths, wander through my favourite woodland, or take myself on a date.

If even this isn't possible, I find small ways to honour my bleed. I wear clothes that make me feel like a goddess (usually in shades of bright red to celebrate my blood), I pour myself fresh hibiscus tea, or I set aside 15 minutes at the end of each day to breathe into my womb and to journal.

You could also create a cocoon-like den for yourself. Smudge the room with smouldering herbs, burn your favourite incense, cosy up with blankets and cushions, meditate, read your favourite books, and enjoy a slice of chocolate cake (see the Chocolate Fudge Cake recipe). You can even create a "womb tent" by draping the room with red fabrics and silks!

What would you like to do for yourself when you next get your period? Write down two or three ideas or intentions, and see this list as your commitment to allow yourself to relax and recharge when you next bleed.

Fatigue shouldn't affect your every day life. If this is the case, seek advice as it could suggest thyroid issues or potential anemia.

Skin

You may notice your skin looks a little more lacklustre, or feels drier than normal. Again, this is completely normal and happens due to our sex hormones plummeting.

To combat this, I tailor and adjust my skincare just as much as I do my diet, my exercise, and my need for rest. If you struggle with dry skin, you might like to consider investing in a good quality hyaluronic acid. I also like to make homemade masks using nourishing ingredients such as honey, yoghurt, and avocado to add TLC to parched skin.

Some women may notice that their skin becomes more irritable and sensitive when they begin their period. This can be due to high amounts of inflammation, so take your time to give your body what it needs to restore.

Cramping

When I was growing up, I struggled with debilitating period cramps. I'd often be writhing in pain, bent over double, or struggling to sleep because my womb would feel like it was about to explode.

Shockingly, studies have shown that up to 93% of women have struggled with dysmennorhoea (the scientific term for period pain) at some point in their lives, particularly during adolescence. So, while not "normal", period pain is incredibly common.

But why does it happen? And what can you do to stop it?

Period pain can be caused by a few things, and it's important to find the root cause. However, cramping is commonly triggered by high oestrogen in relation to progesterone, or high levels of prostaglandins.

Prostaglandins trigger our uterine muscles to contract, resulting in period blood. It's easy to think that we need to rid the body of them, but we actually want just the right amount. Not too much, and not too little.

If you experience regular pain, focus on easing inflammation. This can mean removing inflammatory foods (such as potential allergens, vegetable oils, refined carbohydrates, white bread, alcohol, and trans fats) from your diet, and it can also mean lowering stress (see the Hormone 101 chapter for tips). Omega-3 fatty acids, found in oily fish, walnuts, and chia seeds, are also anti-inflammatory, and may ease period pain.

Ginger, too, is a powerful way to lower inflammation. In fact, some studies show that this warming spice can be just as effective at reducing period pain as anti-inflammatory medications, such as ibuprofen!

Cramp-easing Tricks

Sadly, lowering inflammation is a long-term project, and it will likely take time, and commitment. However, there's plenty you can do to support your beautiful body – and ease period pain – right now. Here are a few tricks:

Legs against the wall

The yoga pose Viparita Karani (aka the less-exciting sounding Legs Against the Wall pose) is a beautiful way to calm and soothe the body, and it can also ease aching or swollen legs and help to lull us into deep sleep. However, it's also known to ease period pain – and it can be done without even rolling out of bed! Other yoga poses which may bring relief include child's pose, seated forward folds, bridge pose, or Shavasana.

Hot water bottle

There's little that's more comforting than a hot water bottle on my period, and it can calm cramping muscles incredibly quickly.

In fact, in Traditional Chinese Medicine (TCM), it's said that women should keep their wombs and feet warm at all times during their bleed to support healthy blood flow. It's also worth pointing out that many women get worse period pain during the cooler winter months (this could be due to lower vitamin D levels).

So, if you experience period pain, see this as your cue: fewer ice baths and bare feet, and more fluffy slippers, blankets, and hot soaks!

Tummy massage

Loving massage is one of my favourite ways to stem period pain. It not only soothes cramping muscles, but it can also support healthy blood flow, and boost natural pain relievers in the body.

To try this for yourself, add a few drops of your favourite essential oils to a carrier oil – such as avocado oil or sweet almond oil – and warm between hands. Next, work it across the belly using gentle circular motions across your abdomen, No heavy-handedness, or pushing down on the tummy. Just loving strokes.

There are lots of sequences you can follow online if you'd like a more guided practice. Just be sure to massage tenderly, with lots of loving energy and thoughts towards your womb. If massaging the tummy feels painful or uncomfortable, stop the practice and try again another time. If discomfort persists, seek advice.

Orgasm

While sex may be the last thing on your mind, orgasm can be a powerful (and fun) way to ease period pain. That's because when we orgasm, our bodies produce pain-relieving endorphins. In fact, in one study in 2000 by Womanizer and Lunette, 90% of women who were given vibrators said that they would recommend orgasm as pain relief. In other words, experiment and have some fun!

If you *do* feel hornier when you're on your period, this is also normal. In fact, some women actually become more orgasmic when they bleed, due to an increase in blood flow.

We may have been taught to have the "ick" over all things messy and all things bloody. Yet, many cultures celebrate period sex as a sacred practice. The key is: do whatever feels good for you.

If pain is persistent or debilitating, please seek support or advice from a Doctor. It could point to Endometriosis, cysts, pelvic inflammatory disease and more.

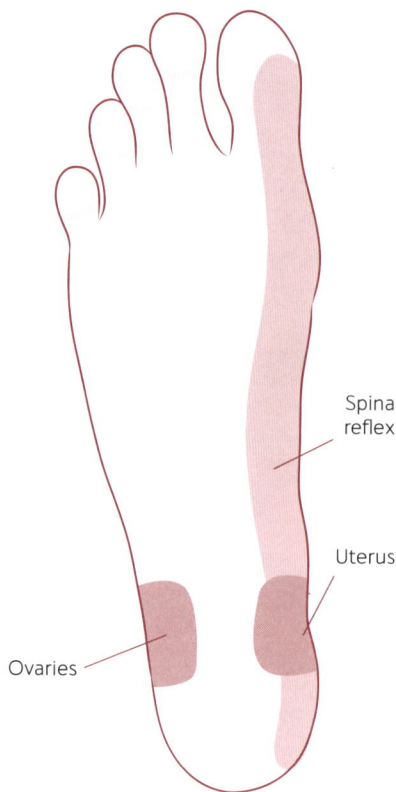

Spina reflex

Uterus

Ovaries

Reflexology
Exercise

✧ • ✧

The following self-reflexology exercise has been written by my incredibly talented friend, Sam Isaacs, to help women who are struggling with period pain. Sam is a reflexologist, aromatherapist, Reiki master, and massage therapist. She works with women from pre-natal to postpartum, through to perimenopausal and beyond. Feel guided and held by her words of wisdom in the following exercise. Reflexology works on the principle that there are pressure points in the feet that correspond with different organs and systems in the body. By working on these, we can restore balance in body, mind, and spirit.

1. As you begin, remember that intuition and senses are heightened during our period. Be gentle with yourself. Tune in to your bodily needs and what unfolds. We are women, wild women, and we are remembering on a soul level who we once were.

2. Anoint your feet with a chosen essential oil, diluted in carrier oil. With flat hands, massage the oil into the feet. Using the backs of your fingers, rhythmically "knuckle" around your ankles. These are the uterus and ovary reflexes and they may feel tender, so ease in.

3. Only go as deep as your body allows. This may look like loving and soothing strokes, or you may like to work deeper.

4. To relax and regulate the nervous system, you can also massage down the instep of the feet. Using your thumb (or fingers if you'd like things to be calmer), massage the joint of the big toe, down to the heel, moving along the bone of the instep. Massage as long as you need to, closing your eyes and concentrating on your breath.

5. Now, take a breath in for a count of four and exhale for a count of eight. Repeat as often as needed, knowing that you are safe, you are loved, and you are protected.

Period Pain

Many women experience more intense pain when their bodies are struggling to release certain emotions, memories, traumas, or even relationships.

The emotional roots

Remember: our period is also a time where we can shed our skins and let go of emotional pain, woundings, traumas, or even limiting beliefs. If you are experiencing period pain, consider asking:

· Is there anything I'm holding onto?

· Is there anything my body is trying to tell me?

How can I support my body in releasing?

Are there any emotions or thoughts/ feelings I might be suppressing?

If you try everything and your period pain persists, it's worth noting that there can be other underlying causes at play. Period pain can be triggered by tight psoas muscles (which play a role in trauma and stress – remember, it's all interconnected!), histamine issues, fibroids, PCOS, pelvic inflammatory disease, adenomyosis, stress or trauma, and the coil.

Endometriosis also commonly causes debilitating period pain, and affects one in ten women. Symptoms include:

· Lower tummy, pelvic or back pain, which worsens during your period (or ovulation)

· Debilitating period pain

· Feeling sick during your period

· Pain during or after sex

· Diarrhoea or chronic constipation before your period

· Heavy bleeding

· Pain when going to the toilet during your period

Endometriosis also means you may struggle during ovulation. For more information, see your doctor and see the Resources section at the end of this book.

Period poops

Believe it or not, period poops are pretty common – especially in connection with IBS. Yet, this symptom isn't talked about enough (likely because bathroom habits tend to be taboo). These bowel changes are usually triggered by a rise in inflammatory prostaglandins. When high, these can stimulate bowel muscles and lead to diarrhoea. The solution? Again, I'd recommend lowering inflammation levels, which we talked about in the cramping section. Many women will also benefit from cutting back on greasy or fried foods, or coffee (sorry). Green tea has been found to lower prostaglandins, so consider switching caffeine for something more calming.

Heavy Bleeding

Many of us carry stories where our menstrual blood has leaked through clothes, stained sofas and bed sheets, or where blood has trickled down our thighs as we play sports. Many of us have been mortified and dashed for the nearest loo. Yet, why? As we've already explored together, our menstrual cycle is a monthly health report and can guide us towards what needs healing. Symptoms are the body's language – and our period blood is no different. In fact, both the colour and the texture of your blood can offer wisdom and insights into the health of your hormones. However, we are all different and I encourage you to work out what is your own normal. As a side note, your blood may look different to the following descriptions if you're on birth control.

What your period blood can mean

If your blood is bright, fresh, cranberry red: This is a sign of a healthy flow. Period blood should be vibrant red in colour, and the consistency of maple syrup – not too thick, but also not too thin. However, if you are experiencing bleeding like this and you're not on your period, please go and see a doctor to be checked over.

If your blood is deep purple: This often indicates excess oestrogen, particularly if accompanied by large clots (small clots are normal), cramps, and heavy bleeding. If this is you, perhaps take a look at your gut and liver health to support healthy hormone elimination (see the Hormone 101 chapter). Deep purple blood with clots can also be common with endometriosis, adenoymosis, or with fibroids, so get it checked out if it concerns you.

If your blood is brown or dark red: Some brown spotting before, or at the end of, your period is normal. However, if it's prolonged, this can suggest that progesterone levels are low. If this occurs, I've found that vaginal steaming (also known as "yoni steaming" – *yoni* is Sanskrit for our female reproductive organs) after ovulation can be helpful in preventing future spotting. However, you'll also want to support your stress (which can also trigger spotting!) and progesterone levels. You may also notice darker brown, almost black blood, at the end of your period. This is normal, and can suggest your uterine lining is being shed slowly. This can also occur if you have a tilted uterus, which affects how quickly you can shed the womb lining.

If your blood is pink: This can indicate that oestrogen is low – common in perimenopause – but can also occur if you have Primary Ovarian Insufficiency or low iron. It can also be blood mixed with cervical fluid, or can mean your body doesn't feel safe. This could be due to intense stress, over-exercising, under-eating, or not eating enough nutrients. Pale pink discharge – particularly when you're not on your period – can also be caused by infection or an underlying condition. As a rule of thumb, it's probably wise to get it checked out by a doctor.

If your blood is grey-tinged in colour, it could be a sign of infection and it's important to seek medical advice. It's also important to note that it's not necessarily a good thing to have a *light* period. If your bleed is very light, lasts only 1–2 days, and your blood is watery in colour (rather than bright red), it could indicate low oestrogen, or a lack of ovulation. However, if you are flooding your pads and tampons, or having to change period products every hour, please seek support from a doctor. If you're unsure or notice any sudden changes, including bleeding when you're not on your period, it's advisable to seek medical advice, since heavy bleeding could also be caused by fibroids and more.

A word on tampons and pads...

I recommend buying the best quality period care you can afford. Unfortunately, many brands of sanitary towels and tampons are treated with harsh chemicals, or may contain potentially harmful heavy metals. Our vaginas and vulvas are highly absorbent, and we should take care with what we wear in close contact with them (this also applies to knickers and body washes!). For this reason, if you can afford it, I'd recommend buying organic cotton tampons or pads, or investing in good quality period pants or menstrual cups. If you struggle with vaginal dryness or discomfort, you might find it helpful to switch from tampons to pads as the absorbent materials in tampons can dry out the vagina. However, the most important thing is that you feel comfortable and confident when using your period products. If this means tampons and moon cups for you, then please continue!

How to Support the Body

As well as honouring our need for rest and warmth, how else can we support our beautiful bodies in the menstrual phase?

Foods

When it comes to nourishing your body, try to tune in to your natural appetite levels. Many women experience a lower appetite during their bleeds, but other women will feel ravenous. Learn to trust in your body and what it's telling you.

In terms of foods to enjoy in abundance, the winter part of your cycle – just like the season – is a time for warming, cosy, comforting foods. Dig into home-cooked soups (if you feel tired, consider meal-prepping them and freezing when energy is high) and stews, and add in warming spices such as ginger or cinnamon. Sip hot herbal teas – nettle is good as it helps to replenish iron levels, while raspberry leaf tea is also perfect for our "Moon Time" – and enjoy earthy root vegetables, such as carrots, potatoes, and squash, to ground your energy.

It's also important to replenish iron. Iron-rich foods include red meat, leafy greens, cacao, and dried apricots. Consider pairing these with a source of vitamin C (such as berries, red peppers, kiwi, broccoli, and lemons) to aid iron absorption.

If you struggle with cramping, you might be interested to know that period pain has been linked to low calcium and vitamin D levels. To increase calcium intake, you can add in leafy greens, organic yoghurt, oranges, and organic tofu. The best way to boost vitamin D will always be through (safe) sun exposure and supplements during the darker months (October to March if you live in the northern hemisphere).

Magnesium, magnesium, magnesium

In an ideal world, none of us would need supplements, *ever*. We'd get all we need to thrive from our diets and the environment around us.

However, we live in far from an ideal world, and many of us are especially low in magnesium. In fact, it's the only supplement I take religiously, and recommend to most women! This is because magnesium can help us with our stress response and sleep, and it can also support blood sugar balance, soothe aching muscles and heads, ease PMS, and reduce period pain.

There are different forms of magnesium which you can take for various needs (for example, magnesium citrate can help with constipation, magnesium sulphate can soothe period pain, and magnesium L-threonate can support memory and cognition). However, a good generic form is magnesium glycinate, which is easily absorbed. This is also helpful if you struggle with stress and overwhelm, PMS, anxiety, or sleep issues. Just be sure to avoid magnesium citrate if you struggle with period poops! For specific concerns, or for guidance on which magnesium supplement is best for you, seek support from a nutritional therapist.

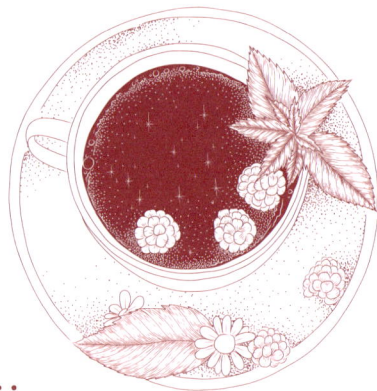

Chocolate
Fudge Cake

✧ • • • • • • • • • • • • • • • • • • • ✧

Speaking of magnesium... One of my favourite ways to boost my intake? Chocolate, chocolate – and more chocolate.

This simple, nourishing chocolate cake is one of my most-loved recipes, and something I make almost every month for my period. It contains no inflammatory ingredients, while sweet potato is naturally sweet and grounding, and cacao is iron-rich and boosts happy hormones. Win, win! Bake this (or, better yet, ask a loved one to bake it for you!), then cut yourself a slice, run a hot bath, and savour every moment.

Ingredients:

Approx 230g (8oz) sweet potato mash (this is made from roughly two medium-sized, cooked sweet potatoes)

200g (7oz) good-quality dark chocolate (70% cacao solids or above)

70g (2½oz) grass-fed, organic butter

95g (3⅓oz) coconut sugar (you can add up to 145g (5oz) if you like things sweeter)

3 tbsp cacao powder

120ml (4oz) milk, or 3 eggs

Pinch of sea salt

1 tsp vanilla

80g (3oz) dark chocolate, finely chopped (optional)

Method:

Preheat your oven to 180°C (350°F) fan. Gently melt together the chocolate and butter in a pan, stirring until silky. Allow to cool for ten minutes, then pour into a blender with the remaining cake ingredients (except the chopped chocolate), and blend until smooth.

Fold in the chocolate chips, then bake in a silicone or loose-bottomed tin (I used a 19cm/7½in silicone tin) for 14–15 minutes, or until cooked on top but gooey inside. Let cool completely, and store in the fridge for the cake to firm up and set.

For an extra treat, drizzle over a homemade ganache by gently melting 125g (4½oz) of dark chocolate with 120ml (4oz) of a milk of your choice.

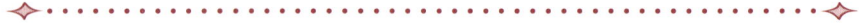

Slow down

We know that our periods are a time to slip into stillness wherever possible, and to slow down. But what do we do about exercise?

For most women, their bleeds – as a time of fatigue and depletion – are the ideal opportunity to take time off movement. Every time I start my period, I ditch exercise completely and rest. Unless it's gentle stretching or walking, I don't do anything. However, it's worth saying that I do this because it feels good for me. If you feel great and strong during your bleed, then listen to yourself, and trust that your body knows best. I'd just encourage you to dial down the intensity a little as you move, since your body will need that energy elsewhere.

Time in nature

When fatigue is high and our bodies have shifted inwards, spending time immersed in Mother Nature is a powerful way to support ourselves. Wandering barefoot across dusty, ochre earth, or treading down on damp grass, can help to ground us when our energies may otherwise float off elsewhere. It can also help us to turn more inwards, to reflect and unravel that deep inner knowing that menstruation brings. Spending more time outdoors can also help to instil some inner calm when we bleed, which is crucial since we can be more sensitive to stress.

If you can't get outside, then bring Mother Nature to you! Dot your house with green plants; add pine essential oil to your diffuser, or create a blend using clary sage, lavender, and peppermint, which medical herbalist Emily Nettleton (see the following herbal bath recipe) says can uplift, reduce stress, and ease cramping; or play the sound of bird song or running water.

Run an Epsom salt bath

How else can you care for your body? Well, we've just learned that boosting our magnesium intake and warming the womb can support our bodies during Moon Time. We also need more time for self-care, to rest, and slow down.

With that in mind, running yourself a soothing Epsom salt bath (rich in magnesium) is the perfect act of self love during your period – and this leads us beautifully onto our final menstrual exercise.

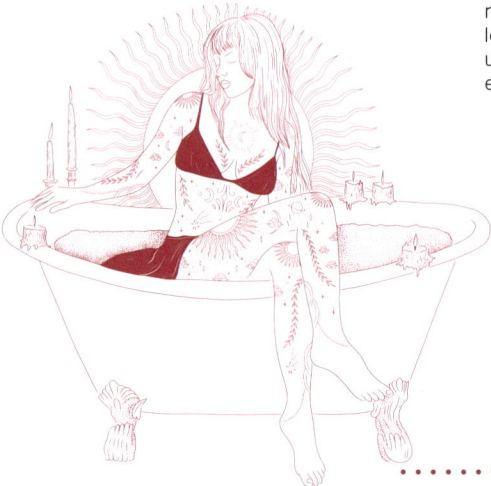

Epsom Salt
Herbal Bath

✧ • • • • • • • • • • • • • • • • • • • ✧

My friend Emily Nettleton, a member of the National Institute of Medical Herbalists, has created this special bath blend to help us to relax, and to ease any period pain we may experience. If you don't experience pain, you can simply use the Epsom salts for a magnesium boost!

Herbalism is a powerful and ancient practice, and can act as a bridge between modern western worlds and ancient ones. As a medical herbalist, Emily also sells her own range of teas and remedies, organises herbal workshops, and leads guided walks in her community. She is one of the most knowledgeable healers I know, so please look out for her activities and follow her on social media!

Ingredients:

95g (3⅓oz) Epsom salts

1 tbsp dried cramp bark

1 tbsp dried raspberry leaf

1 tbsp ground ginger

Optional: Make this bath a ritual by adding in your favourite essential oils, or popping in crystals, such as rose quartz for self love.

Method:

In a small bowl, mix together the salts and herbs. Run a bath to your desired temperature, then pour in the salts. Swirl and combine until they've dissolved, then submerge yourself in the water (healing in itself!). Relax, unwind, and enjoy.

What's Happening Emotionally?

Our bodies aren't the only things which ebb and flow through our cycle. As women, our brains are also cyclical, and our moods can also change. Here's what you might notice in this phase...

Need to withdraw

With hormones at a low point, many women experience an urge to withdraw. Even if you're normally a fluttering social butterfly, your energy will likely shift into a more inward and introspective state. You may crave more alone time, or find yourself longing to slip into stillness and silence. This is partly to allow our bodies to replenish and heal, but it's also Mother Nature's cue to take time out. In doing so, we can understand all that needs releasing, and listen to our inner voice so that we can gather wisdom for the rest of our cycle.

Questions for you to ponder include: how can you honour this need for stillness? How can you allow yourself this time? This can be difficult – particularly if you're a mama to young children. However, it's crucial for your health and your spirit that you carve out some time – even if it's only five minutes – to allow yourself to journey inwards.

Stress-sensitive

Many women find they are more sensitive to stressors in this phase. You might feel more on edge or jumpier than normal, and you might also feel snappy – particularly if you don't get time to yourself, or if you're surrounded by bright lights or the hum of people. Wherever you can, build calming, mood-regulating practices into your period days, and I promise you will find your bleed a much gentler time. Try box breathing (see the Nervous System section, in the Hormone 101 chapter), inhale soothing scents (such as lavender or chamomile), take a break from the on-screen thrillers, and try to protect your energy at all costs.

Challenging views

Our periods can also be tricky because we are surrounded by toxic views. Many women don't feel able to openly talk about their bleeds, or how they're feeling, which leads to us squashing and burying things that need to be unleashed.

Sadly, when we're immersed in a world that holds our periods in a shameful light, those same views can also start to bleed into our own thoughts – even if we don't realise it.

Wherever you can, get curious about how you feel towards your period. Ask yourself questions without judgement (it's OK if you loathe your period!). Tell your loved ones how you're feeling, and don't be afraid to ask for what you need.

Many women also find that there's a lot of power in reclaiming their menstrual blood. After spending most of our lives being made to feel dirty for our periods, seeing your blood in a new light can be a powerful shift.

Two Rituals

If you'd like to, your period is the perfect time to create blood magic and reclaim your body as your own. You can explore what works for you, and even research some rituals online, but here are two ideas:

Anoint yourself

Use a small dot of menstrual blood to anoint your third eye, in the centre of your forehead between your eyebrows. As you anoint yourself, you can speak out an affirmation to yourself. Choose whichever words come to you, but you could say: "I am powerful, and my blood and body are sacred". You can also use it to anoint your other feminine centres – your heart and your womb. Traditionally, the Hindu bindi is thought to be a symbolic celebration of menstrual blood.

Plant fertiliser

Unbeknown to many, menstrual blood is a powerful plant fertiliser. I can vouch for this: each of my plants (and I have many – I am the epitome of Crazy Plant Lady) that I have watered with my blood has gone on to blossom, bloom and thrive, towering above the plants that I haven't fed my blood. It is also a powerful way to connect to Mother Earth – a nod to the fact that, like the Earth, we are also cyclical. Women are the keepers of life and death, birth and rebirth.

As a word of warning: please dilute your blood with water before feeding to the plants. If you don't use a moon cup, you can collect your blood by free bleeding into a jar or pot, or by soaking pads and tampons in water.

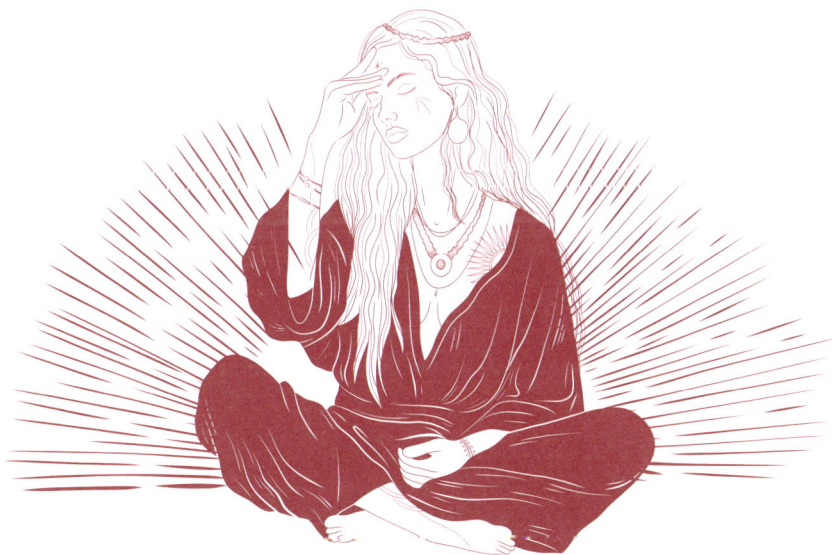

Winter's Super Powers

Don't conclude that your period is a time full of things you *shouldn't* do. Yes, your body may feel more fatigued and tired. And, yes, you may feel a huge pull to burrow yourself beneath your duvet and hibernate for the next few days. But, your period (in fact, your entire cycle) is a super power. Here are just a few of the reasons why your period makes you a Bad Ass...

Connection

Our period is a reminder that we are One with all life. Just like the moon, the Earth and the seasons, women cycle and spiral through life. We hold the cycles of life (of death and rebirth) within our wombs, and we move through them with each bleed. This in itself is a miraculous and wondrous thing. A woman is not a fixed creature: she moves and cycles effortlessly through life, moving as one with the plants, animals, trees and water around her. She is Gaia, or Mother Earth, embodied, and she connects us to our ancestors and to all that lives and has lived.

Shed and release

As we bleed, we're called to let go of toxic relationships and situations. We're called to release limiting thoughts and beliefs. And we're also asked to let traumatic memories or emotions dissolve from the body.

Goddess, your bleed is asking you to transform – and it's asking you to transform into your most powerful self. This becomes ever more possible when we learn to trust in our Crone wisdom and energies.

To do this, I imagine these things leaving my body as I free bleed onto the Earth. If that's not for you, you could write them down on paper as a ritual, before (carefully and symbolically) burning it. Alternatively, you could stand beneath the shower, allowing the water to purify and cleanse your skin.

If it seems scary to let go of things, that's OK: start gently, and start small. You could even work with the guidance of a therapist or a coach, if you feel the need for it.

However, remember: our womb has the power to regenerate every single month, and you too hold this power.

Questions to ponder:

- As your body sheds its uterine lining, what emotional debris would you like to shed and release this cycle? What are you holding onto that no longer serves you?

- What do you want from life, or from your next cycle? What do you need to do to be able to achieve this?

- Are you experiencing any physical symptoms as you bleed? Could these have emotional or spiritual roots?

Crone wisdom

Just like the Crone – our winter archetypal woman – a woman bleeds wisdom. Ancient communities knew this. In fact, male shamans were thought to ingest period blood to enhance their own powers. In other communities, women retreated when they bled so that they could enjoy stillness and gather wisdom for their tribes.

Your primal wisdom and energy run deep, and your bleed makes you radically, powerfully charged. You are an unstoppable, all-knowing force, so take some time to harness and cultivate this energy so that you can live your dream life. Carve out some quiet time so that your cauldron can bubble and simmer with deep wisdom. Journal and free write, paint or sing, meditate, or do tarot or card pulls to tap into your subconscious. If you struggle to access this wisdom, then think of other ways you can access Crone energy. You could pray to the Crone goddesses (such as Hecate, Kali, or the demi-goddess Circe), or drape yourself in red, the colour of our blood and the priestess.

But above all else: trust in yourself, and trust in whatever wisdom comes to you in this phase. Don't doubt yourself, and use it to start your next cycle – your next chapter – afresh.

Quick reaction times

Curiously, one of our super powers in this phase is also heightened cognitive abilities. In fact, new studies – released as I write this book – have shown that, even though women feel more depleted during their bleed, their reaction times shoot up. The study was conducted on women who took part in tests that mimicked team sports, and it also showed that women tended to make fewer errors during their bleed. While I'd always advise against using this as evidence that you can go full throttle on your period, it does shine a light on the toxic messaging that women are less than, or inferior, when on their periods.

Girl, you're a freaking superhero!

A Final Word...

No matter how you feel about your menstrual cycle, I hope that this has helped you to recognise that there is another way. That you are wild, powerful, and untameable – and that we all have access to deep, primal knowledge in our wombs.

Goddess, your period is your super power. It's *the* super power. And it's here to lead the way to your happiest, healthiest life.

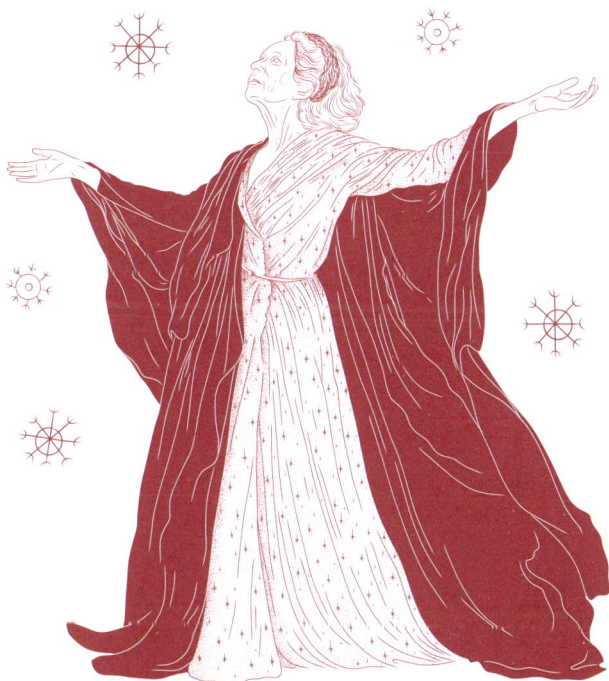

Spring

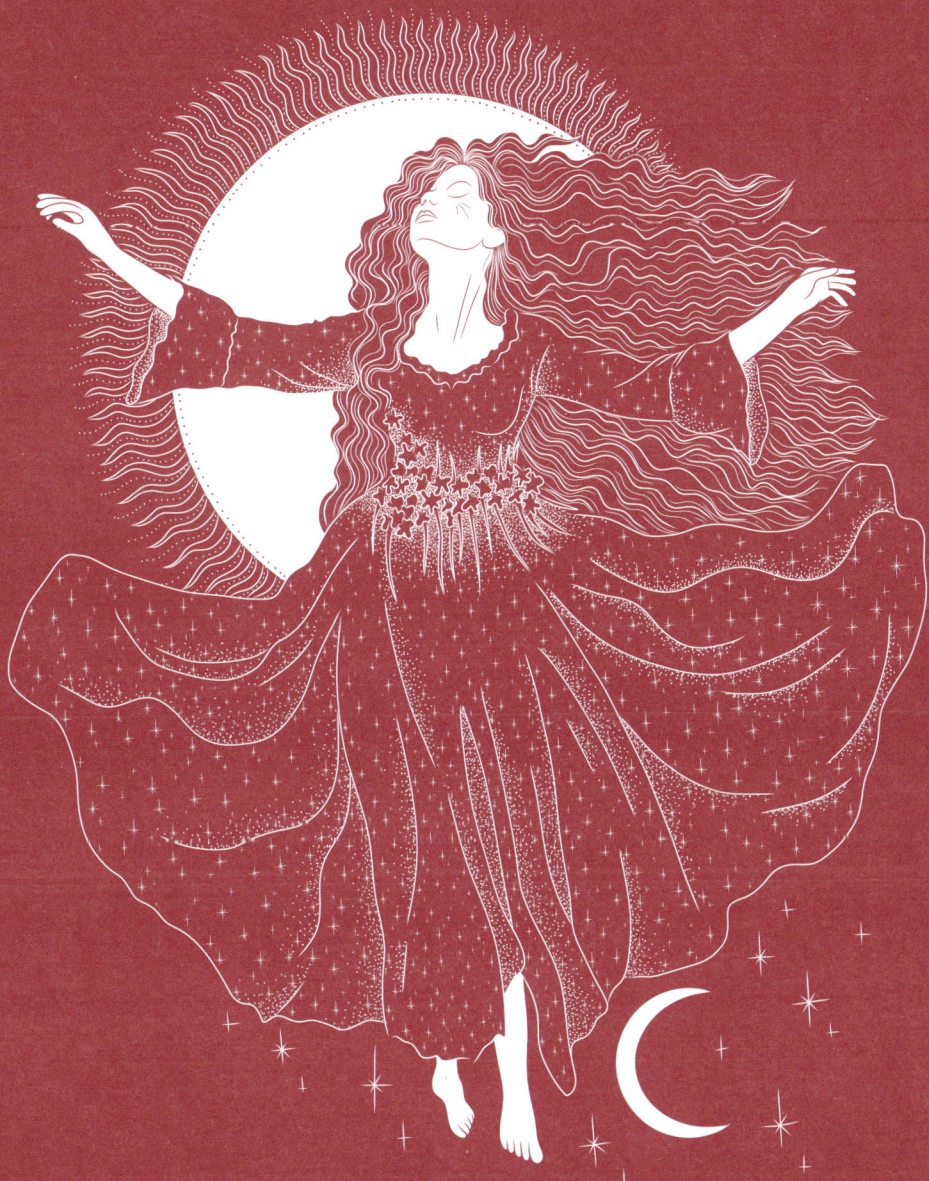

Follicular Phase, aka Spring

As we close the door on our powerful Crone, we welcome in the lighter, fresher, more childlike energy of the Maiden. Our follicular phase, known as "Inner Spring", can be a welcome relief (and a gulp of blossom-scented air) for the many women who struggle with their periods.

Days 6–12 (approx) of your cycle

Archetype:
Maiden

Moon phase:
Waxing moon

"When we dim our light to make others feel more comfortable, the whole world gets darker."

Dr Christiane Northrup, *Dodging Energy Vampires*

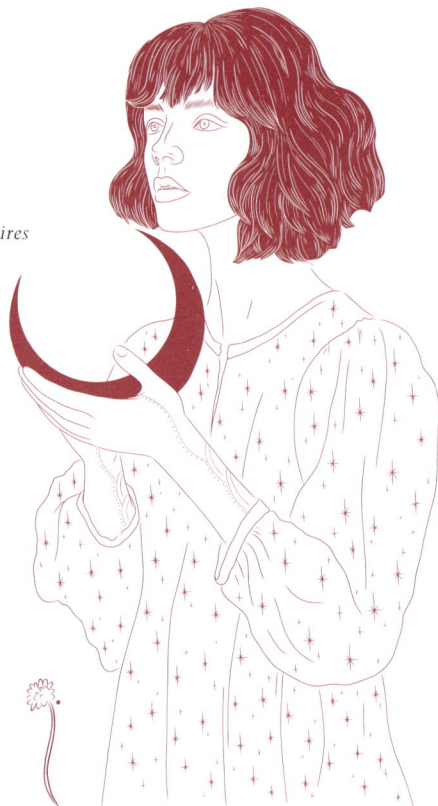

Following winter, which can cloak our bodies in a foggy veil, the follicular phase seems wondrous. We look at the world with a new energy, with childlike awe. We are Sleeping Beauty, awakening to soft-petalled kisses.

Just like the season of spring, this too is the menstrual phase of rebirth. As we enter it, we pave the way for new beginnings. We throw open the windows and welcome in the warm breeze, and we stand back and admire the tender green shoots we've encouraged to sprout from the frozen earth.

There's also a sense of growing confidence and energy. Of curiosity and learning, of dreaming, creating and manifesting. It's here that we can unearth our Inner Child and infuse them with love through play, fun, and time to be silly.

Of course, for some women, the introverted energy of our bleed – which gives us permission to squirrel ourselves away – can feel like a safety net. Poking your nose out from the menstrual cave and preparing to rejoin the world can feel a bit overwhelming.

Yet, whichever line you sit on, the follicular phase has its own remarkable powers. Let's settle down and learn the spring magic together.

What's Happening Physically?

As our bodies slowly creep away from that heavy menstrual energy, our Inner Child begins to reawaken. This is related to those hormonal ebbs and flows – our brain, our energy, our mood, our libido can all be impacted by our cycle.

After our hormone levels were at their lowest point during winter, things are now starting to build and grow. As our bleed ends, oestrogen – the shiny, sociable hormone – starts to rise after its winter slumber.

At the same time, follicle stimulating hormone (more easily remembered as FSH) rises. This stimulates the ovarian follicles, encouraging the preparation of an egg for ovulation.

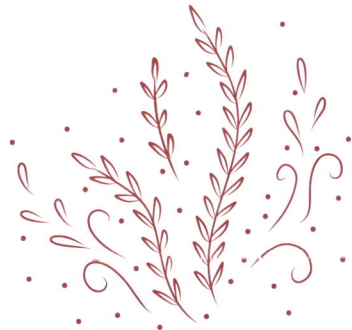

What Else Might You Notice?

Energy

The further you move into your follicular phase, the more you'll likely feel your energy start to rise and build. You may feel more vibrant, less tired – and your zest for life will (hopefully) return. After feeling fatigued and depleted during our periods, it can be tempting to go gung-ho and throw ourselves into every social meeting, every project, and every opportunity. Yet, as a word of caution: try not to over-do it in this phase, especially before your energy peaks. When we do too much too soon, we can burn ourselves out for the rest of our cycle. Instead, ease yourself in gently. Take baby steps before you start to re-emerge into the full sun.

Discharge

Following your bleed, you may have very little discharge. However, as you move through the follicular phase, you might notice an increase in cervical mucus on your knickers. Our natural wetness increases as oestrogen rises, before becoming stickier, stretchier, and clearer as we near ovulation. I've spoken to many women who have been concerned or alarmed by this discharge. However – likely because our vaginas and vulvas are a mystifyingly taboo topic – they're too scared to ask about this increase in wetness.

Cervical mucus, or discharge, is produced by the cervix (what I like to call the gatekeeper to our womb), which is housed at the roof of the vagina and the base of the womb. Both the texture and the amount of discharge can change with our hormones, and it works to keep our vagina clean (yes, your vagina is self-cleaning!) and stop potentially harmful substances from entering the womb. Our discharge also helps sperm to travel upwards to potentially fertilise an egg.

So, as long as your discharge is white, creamy or clear in colour, doesn't itch or burn, isn't thick or cottage-cheese-like in texture and doesn't smell, it's likely completely normal – and healthy.

Appetite

If your appetite didn't drop during your period (although, side bar: it doesn't always, mine never does and I would gladly eat my own arm most periods), then it's likely you'll feel it shift here. Many women find their appetites decrease during Inner Spring. Our insulin sensitivity is also much better here, so you may notice an urge to eat and enjoy lighter, fresher foods and meals.

Skin

You know you've hit Inner Spring when you look in the mirror and notice a gorgeous glow, and an extra sparkle and shine in your eyes.

Oestrogen plays an important role in collagen production, so our skin tends to look dewy and radiant as this hormone rises. You can support this healthy, fresh face by exfoliating a few times during the spring part of your cycle, removing dead skin cells and increasing cell regrowth. I also like to enhance my glow by using a vitamin C-based serum.

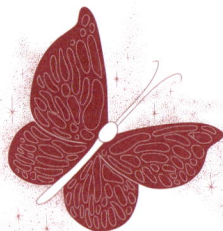

What's Happening Emotionally?

As our hormones start to build and rise, our spring Maiden dances in, bringing with her lighter, more joyful and playful emotions. Glimmers of joy may start to seep back into our lives, while our Inner Child may see the world with a renewed sense of curiosity and wonder. Here's what else we may experience in spring...

Social butterfly re-emerges

As we creep closer to ovulation, the inwards energy of menstruation starts to spin and dance, before spiralling outwards. In spring, you'll likely feel more sociable, more energetic, and more willing to step out into the world. Similarly, as testosterone rises, most women will also start to feel more confident and daring, and your libido may start to make an appearance once again.

Dreamer

After diving into our deep inner psyches when on our periods, many women find that goals and dreams – either life-long or short-term – bubble to the surface in this phase.

With your body starting a fresh new chapter, you may also feel an urge to lay the groundwork for new beginnings. You may throw your face to the sky and daydream and wonder as you watch clouds float by. Or you may have clarity about goals you want to set, and ideas you want to birth into this world. Whatever it is, let your rational mind go – and let your daydreamer run wild!

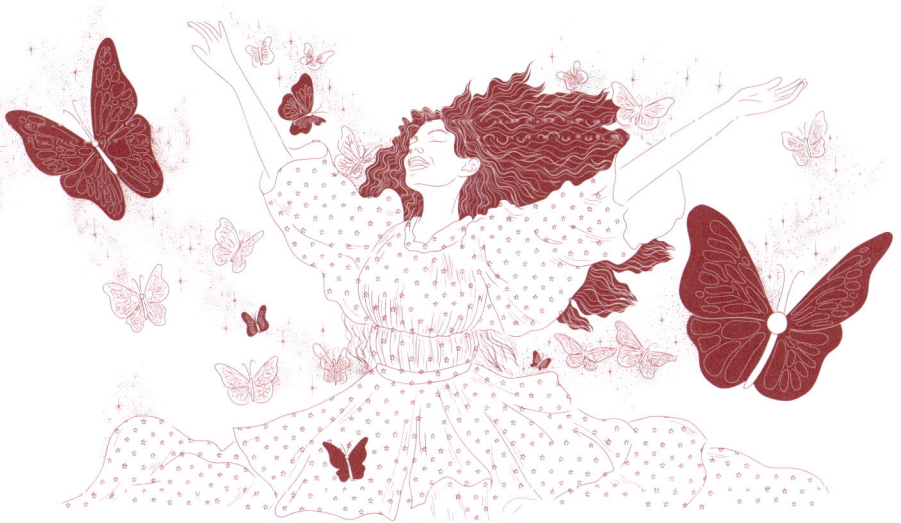

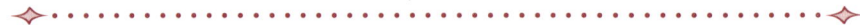

Playfulness

When I was a little girl, I'd spend summer holidays swimming beneath the surface of shimmering pools. As damp tendrils of golden hair fell onto sun-kissed skin, I'd glide through the water, dipping and diving, pretending I was a mermaid.

Back home, I'd pass time crushing summer berries. The inky juices stained half-moon nails as I made potions, wine, or food for fairies. My head firmly in the clouds – or perhaps rooted in reality, depending on how you see it – I'd also dance around circles of mushrooms, and lay down painted acorn cups for fairies to use as bowls.

My childhood was passed with one foot in this world, one foot out. Yet, somewhere along the way, I lost my glimmering, childlike wonder. My playful, joyful Maiden became submerged beneath a shroud of responsibility, exam pressures, and "Real Life".

I know I'm not alone, and I know that, for many women, the playful part of this phase is one we struggle to embrace. Yet, we need to reclaim our Inner Child so that we can tap into spring-like joy, and rediscover our spark and love for life. If you've lost your playful energy, then your follicular phase is the perfect place to re-discover it!

A combination of traumas and repressed emotions mean that I still find this difficult, but I'm getting there. My Inner Child comes out when I leap on the supermarket trolley and glide (or fly!) down the aisle, or when I roll across damp summer grass with my youngest boy, and hurtle down sand dunes on holiday.

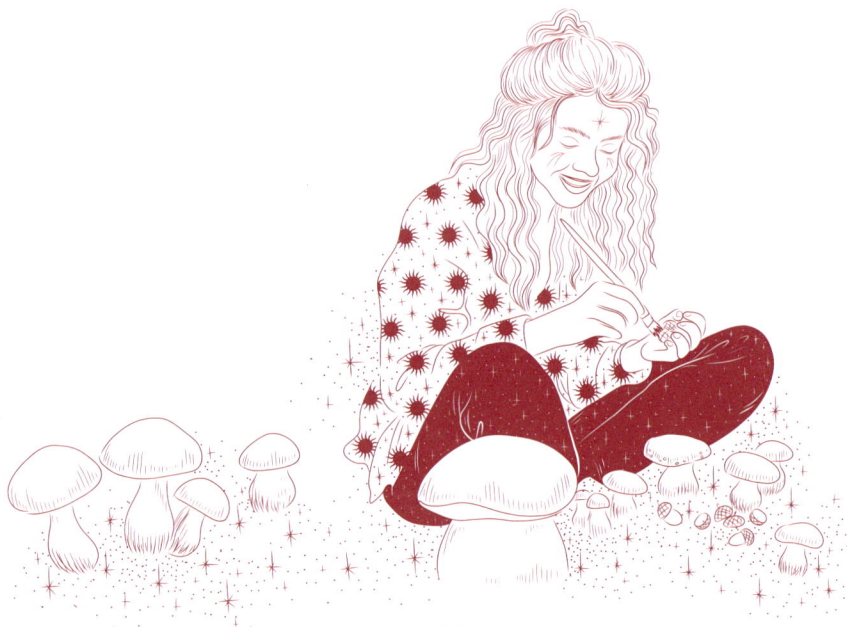

If you struggle to rediscover playfulness, here are some questions to contemplate, to sit with in your womb, or to journal:

- How does your Inner Child feel right now? What does she need?
- If you allowed your Inner Child to play, what would you do? Do you feel you're able to play and be silly?
- How can you pepper this playful energy into your day?
- What did you most love to do as a child, before the outside world had a chance to shape it?
- Do you still do it? If not, why not?
- What last sparked your inner joy and curiosity?
- Is there anything new your Inner Child would like you to try?

Set goals

Fun fact: I never set resolutions or goals at new year. To me, it's always felt odd to reach for the stars when the world around is so bare. Instead, spring has always felt like true new year (fun fact: spring actually is new year in many cultures, for example in Iran), and it's in this season that I set my intentions.

Similarly, the spring phase of your cycle is the time to dream big, and set yourself some goals. You might like to plan goals for your year ahead, or you may like to think a little smaller and set some goals for this menstrual cycle.

Whatever goals you want to achieve, tap into that rising testosterone and embrace your growing confidence – don't be afraid to dream big. Trust me, the possibilities are endless.

When you're next in your follicular phase, I'd like you to think about all the things you learned about yourself in winter. Now, ask: what three goals would I like to set right now? Write them down as your commitment to yourself.

Essential oils

If you struggle to tap into the light-hearted energy of spring, or if you're still feeling heavy and sluggish after winter, essential oils can be a powerful way to shift your energy. Try the Essential Oil Diffuser Recipe that follows to put some spring into your spring.

Practice gratitude and wonder

One of the most beautiful qualities of the Maiden is her curiosity and awe for even the simplest of things. She sees magic in the minute, shimmers of awe in the every day, and glimmers of joy in the things that adults don't notice – a line of insects scurrying across sunbaked earth, for example. An arc of stars, pin pricks against a velvet backdrop. The simple, sweet joy of the first lick of ice cream on a sizzling summer day.

This is the perfect phase for rediscovering the joy and wonder in life, and recognising the magic that lies abundant in the world. Commit to noticing what's around you. Go glimmer hunting. Take a mindful walk. Keep a gratitude journal at the end of the day, and list three things you're grateful for – no matter how big or small. Bonus: gratitude is also proven to lower stress, and boost health.

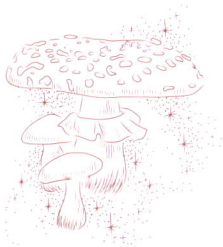

Essential Oil
Diffuser Recipe

✦ • • • • • • • • • • • • • • • • • • • ✦

My dear friend Emily Nettleton, whom you met in the last chapter, has crafted this divine essential oil recipe to help you to embrace the magic of spring.

This beautiful blend will help to invigorate your senses, and can harmonise your body's rising energy. These oils also stimulate the mind, enhance mood, and support hormonal balance. They also work through the limbic system to boost spirits and cultivate a sense of optimism.

Combine the following essential oils in your diffuser:

3 drops of geranium

3 drops of lemon

3 drops of rosemary

Sit back, and enjoy the uplifting aroma. If you like, you can use this recipe to help you to set goals, or to enhance your creativity. Whatever you use it for, let yourself savour and enjoy it!

Go on a
Mindful Walk

◆ • • • • • • • • • • • • • • • • • • ◆

How often do you take the simple things for granted?
Or forget to find the joy in the every day?

So often I walk my dog, Cato, as a chore. I see it as Another Thing to Do, something to tick off and get done quickly – and I end up resenting it. Yet, when I slow things down, when I stop to smell sprays of colourful sweet peas, or watch the bees as they hum and buzz, it becomes one of my favourite things about the day. It quickly shifts dog walking from a stressor to a glimmer.

So, your next exercise is to go on a mindful walk. It's simple to do, and you can do it anytime, anywhere. All that I ask is that you give it a go, and you aim to do it at least twice during this phase.

1. Pick somewhere you'd like to walk to. It can be an old haunt, or somewhere new. Try to let yourself feel some excitement for this place that you're going to explore.

2. As you walk and wander, connect to your breath. Take big breaths in through the nose, and let your belly rise and expand. Exhale any stress or tension away, through the mouth with a gentle "ahhhh".

3. Get curious about how you're feeling. What's your energy like today? How does your body feel? Are there any areas of tightness or tension, or do you feel free and relaxed? Ask these questions without judgement – just curiosity. Acknowledge whatever you're feeling, and move on.

4. Now, start to notice things around you. What can you see that you may not ordinarily notice? What colours can you spot? What insects or animals can you find? Are there any sounds you can hear? What can you see that brings beauty to your day?

5. If it feels safe to do, sit down and immerse yourself deeper in this spot. How does it feel to be here? Can you let your body soften into the Earth beneath you until you root into the ground and become one with Mother Nature?

6. Thank the place you've visited. If you feel called to, leave a small offering – such as an apple – for the fairy and land spirits around you. As you walk home, stay curious about how you feel. Has anything shifted or changed since you started walking?

Try something new

Tap into that youthful, vibrant energy by trying something new. As your body embraces a more playful quality, you might even like to try something that you might otherwise be mortified by: go to a belly dancing class, roll down a hill covered in daisy chains, or prance around the garden with a homemade flower crown perched on your head.

You could also sign up to learn a new language, buy or borrow a book on a subject you've always found fascinating, or visit somewhere completely new. Delve into new cultures, cook a new cuisine, or sign yourself up to a class at the gym. It could even be as simple as taking a new path to work. Whatever it is, let your curiosity shine through!

How to Support the Body

Exercise

You're going to get so tired of me saying this, but: listen to your body, and tune into your energy levels! When you finish your period, your energy may still be fairly low. Let yourself rest if you need to, or do some slow and gentle movement.

As energy rises, you might find you're able to push your body a little more. Cortisol levels also tend to be lower in this phase and in ovulation, so you may find you're able to ramp up the intensity and push yourself a little harder.

You could plan an outdoor adventure and go hiking, or rock climbing, or you might want to harness your playful energy with skipping or Zumba. Some studies have shown that you might feel stronger now, with some women experiencing greater increases in muscle strength. This means that it could be a brilliant phase to embrace your inner strength and get weight training!

Whatever it is, listen to your body!

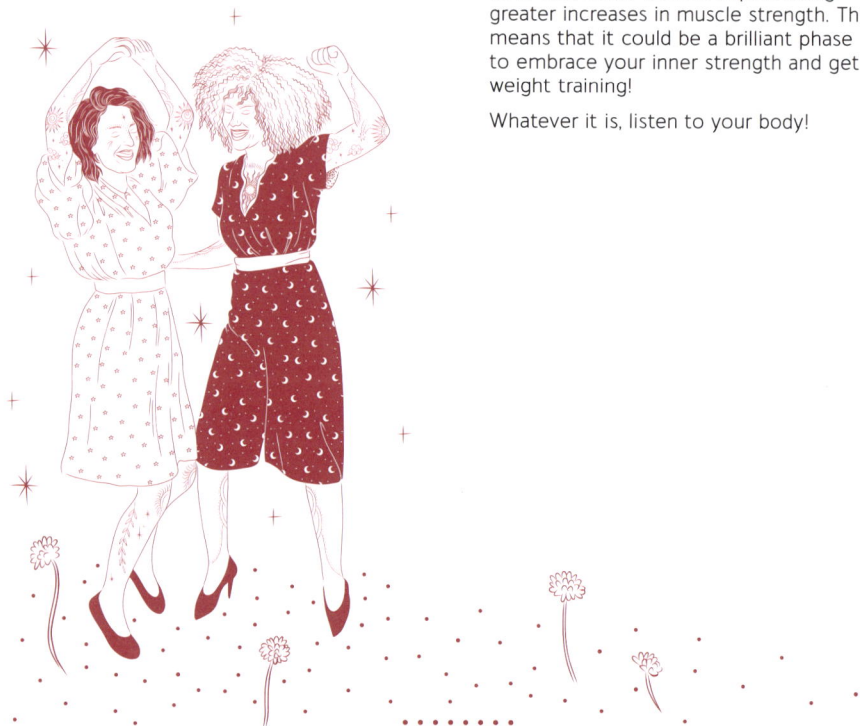

Food

Embracing and enjoying certain foods in the follicular phase can mean we pave the way for a healthier cycle and less painful bleed.

As you leave your period behind, continue to replenish your body with plenty of iron-rich foods, paired with a side of vitamin C.

As we've already discovered, many women experience a lower appetite at this time – and often have a higher tolerance for stress. For this reason, if you want to try intermittent fasting, I'd recommend embracing it in your follicular phase. However, I wouldn't advise fasting in any other phase of your cycle – particularly if you struggle with hormonal imbalances.

Next, aim to embrace gorgeous, healthy fats, such as avocado, eggs, nuts, and extra virgin olive oil. If, like me, you grew up in the toxic 90s and 00s era of low-fat dieting (flashbacks to the me of that age, mainlining family bags of marshmallows because they were "low fat", and then wondering why my periods were painful, my skin so inflamed, and my moods and weight so haywire), this can seem counter-intuitive.

Yet, I promise you: we need plenty of healthy fats in our diets. Healthy fats are one of the building blocks of our hormones, and they are crucial in helping us to thrive! Similarly, we also need plenty of protein for the correct synthesis of hormones. Since we may have a lower appetite in this phase, embrace lean proteins as you move deeper into your follicular phase – think foods such as chicken, prawns, or organic tofu. You'll still need to eat carbs, but you may find you're able to eat far less than your body craved during your period.

As oestrogen continues to rise, it's also important to help our bodies to eliminate excess hormones. Remember: soaring levels of oestrogen (particularly if paired with low progesterone) can cause us all kinds of problems further down the line. This means our spring Maidens can benefit from fibre-rich foods (although tread with caution if you struggle with bloating), as well as foods that can support our gut. In particular, I like to enjoy fermented foods, such as kefir, kimchi, kombucha, natural yoghurt, and sourdough.

You can also add in phytoestrogens here, which mimic the effects of oestrogen in the body. While these foods can support healthy oestrogen production, they also work to regulate high levels of oestrogen. These foods include red clover, ground flax, and pumpkin seeds.

Finally, as your body starts its work in preparing an egg, try to eat lots of antioxidant-rich foods. These foods – such as berries and dark, leafy greens – are important for follicular and egg health. Pomegranates and eggs are also thought to improve egg quality.

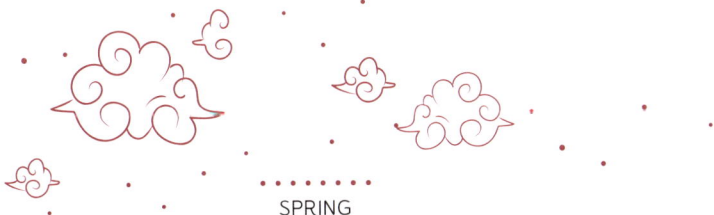

Spring's Super Powers

The enchantment and wonder of our Inner Spring phase makes this season full of joyful magic. With our Maiden in the driver's seat, we're able to let our playfulness and imagination take over. Thanks to a high sense of trust and new beginnings – and also the power of creativity at our fingertips – this is where we can manifest and plant the seeds of our deepest dreams.

Embrace joy

Far too often, we're bombarded with doom and gloom. We open our phones and mindlessly scroll to news of wars, suffering, and pain. While it's important to be aware of what's around us and what's going on in the world, it's also important to remember the joy in life.

In this fizzy, shimmering phase, it's easier to embrace the joy and see the good in life. In fact, many women – especially those who struggle with their periods, PMS, or ovulation pain – can find that this is the only phase of their cycle where they truly thrive. If this is you, then I'd advise you to seek support: you don't deserve to feel at your worst for 75% of the month. In fact, if you do feel this way, then it may (but not always!) suggest underlying issues, such as PCOS, endometriosis, or thyroid problems.

However you feel for the rest of your cycle, your real super power here lies in finding life's glimmers. While outside stressors may come and go (life, after all, happens for us all, no matter our menstrual phase), and our expectations should never be to be calm and happy 100% of the time (we need to feel our emotions – *all* of them – to be truly alive), you'll find it far easier to dust yourself down and embrace the silver linings here.

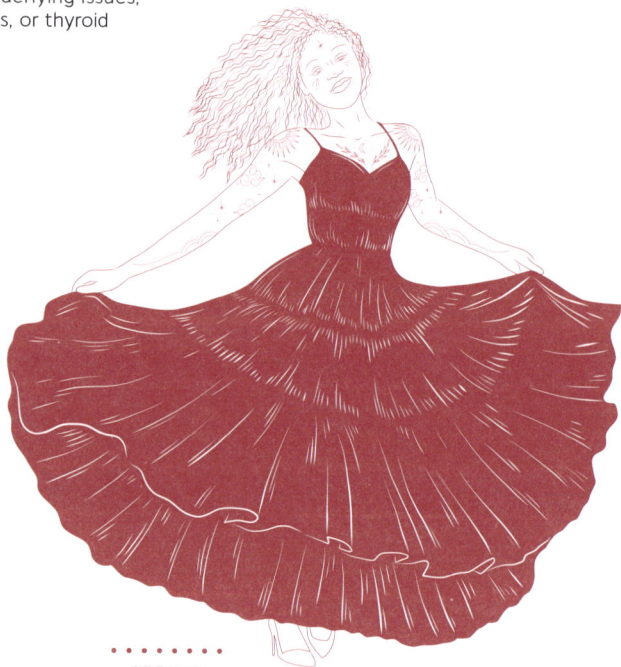

For this reason, consciously spend time living in the moment when you enter spring. Belly laugh until you snort or cry. Leap and dance about and be silly. Tell ridiculous jokes. Skip instead of walk. Hula hoop or blow bubbles. Stop and smell beautiful flowers.

Let yourself find your spark.

Brainstorm and manifest

Another of your super powers? Brainstorming and manifesting all that your Maiden heart most desires. As we enter into this new beginning, it's the perfect time for channelling the accompanying shift in hormones for your own good. New ideas flow easily here – imagination can rise during the follicular phase – so take advantage, sit down, and have a brainstorming session! If you are a more visual person, you might like to create a vision board of your ideas.

This is where we plant the seeds of our deepest desires. After releasing everything that no longer served us during our period, now is the time to ask: what is it we actually want to call in? What are we being called to create? What steps do we need to take towards finding our purpose?

You'll also find it far easier to surrender and trust in the process in this phase.

Bay leaf manifestation spell

If you want to embrace your inner witch, you could even try a simple manifesting spell. I like to use bay leaves for manifestation. Not only are bay leaves spiritually associated with attracting positive energy and shunning negative energy, but they're also cheap and easy to find.

To start manifesting, take a pencil and write what you want to call in onto a bay leaf. Alternatively, write a list of all that you want to welcome in, and place it beneath your pillow at night.

As a tip, write as if your wish has already happened – and write in as much detail as possible. For example, "I am earning £5,000 a month by helping my dream clients to achieve health and happiness".

Now, let yourself envision this happening. Picture it in your head, let yourself feel the emotions and joy it brings. What difference does this make to your life? What do you do differently? Does it change your health?

Now, very carefully, and as safely as possible (I like to do this in my bathroom or outdoors), set fire to the bay leaf. As it starts to smoke, imagine that your dreams are winging their way into the ether, into the universe, ready to be transformed

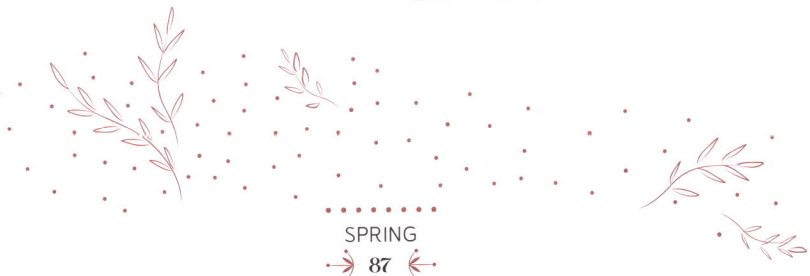

Creativity

Rising oestrogen can also boost mental sharpness and creativity. Spring means we're preparing to birth and create new life. This can come in the form of a fertilised egg, but it can also mean creative endeavours, new projects, or new businesses.

In fact, when women don't harness their creativity, or when they shut it tightly away, it can cause symptoms or trigger health issues. For example, our ovaries are linked to our creative powers, and I've seen many ovarian cysts in women who haven't been able to birth or create the things that they desire.

A gentle reminder too: creativity looks different for us all. You don't have to be a painter, a photographer, or a poet to be creative. Creativity can also take the form of planning your business's social media content, recording a podcast episode, keeping a daily journal, singing and dancing (even if just for yourself!), cooking a new meal, or playing the alchemist and creating homemade bath salts using your favourite essential oils and flowers from the garden.

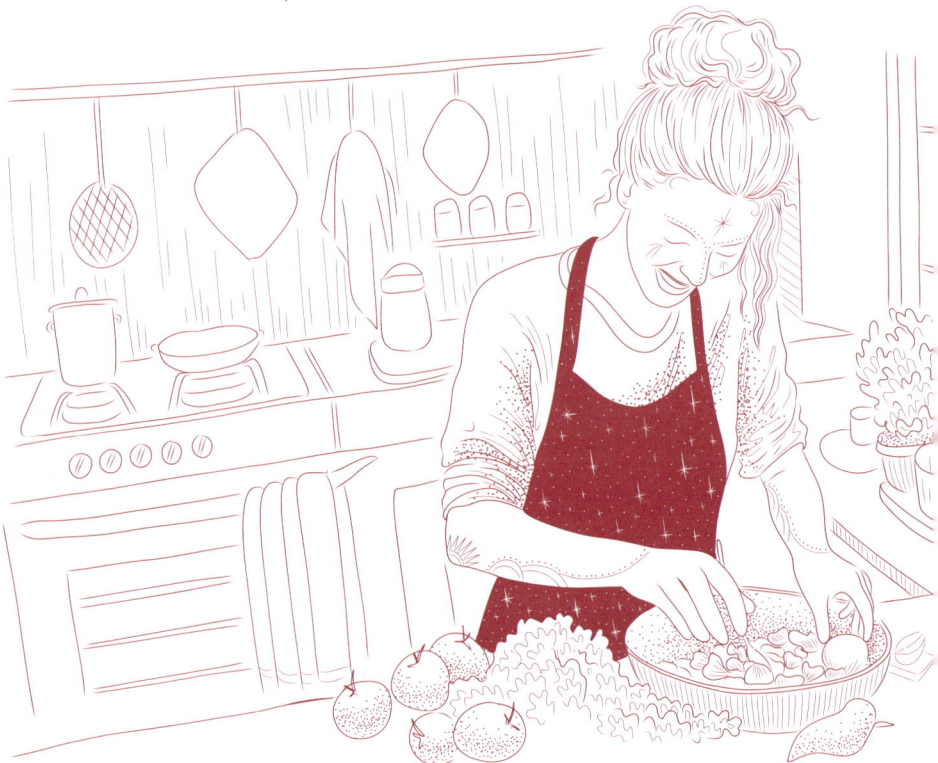

So, as you cycle through Inner Spring, ask yourself:

- What do you feel the urge to create this cycle?
- What are your creative gifts?

If you're not sure where to begin, are there any things you used to enjoy as a child that you could be called to rediscover?

If I'm struggling to create, I also find getting outdoors helps me to focus and be inspired. In fact, as I tap tap tap away at my laptop to write this, I'm currently sitting in my garden, sun blazing down, birds chirruping away, and I'm feeling happy, focused, and completely inspired.

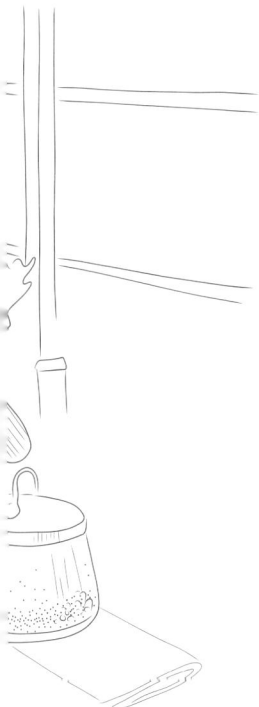

Self Love

Since it's far easier to see the positives, many women find it easier to truly love and accept themselves in this phase. You'll likely find that this only grows the closer you get to ovulation. In fact, after wanting to hide away in your menstrual phase while picking at every last imagined flaw on your goddess face, chances are you now feel cute, beautiful, and every bit like the colourful butterfly emerging from the chrysalis.

As women, so many of us have been taught to neglect or abandon ourselves. To loathe our bodies and faces, and to focus on our flaws. Yet, as we've come to learn, each one of our bodies – just as they are – is an altar. We deserve to be able to surrender to love, and we deserve to be able to celebrate ourselves as beautiful.

This isn't arrogance – it's our birthright.

That's why this is the perfect phase to enjoy the next and final spring exercise: a beautiful Body Blessing. However, this can be done anytime, anywhere, and at any point in your cycle when you feel a need to give yourself some love.

Body Blessing
Exercise

❖ • • • • • • • • • • • • • • • • • • • ❖

Use this experience to honour your body, to help yourself
feel into and experience it in all its magic, and to help you
to connect to your sensuality, wonder, and beauty.

1. Create yourself a sacred space where you won't be disturbed. This will likely look different for all of us, but it could be in front of your altar, or it could be in a quiet, peaceful room at home. I like to burn candles (red or pink represent self love, while white represents innocence and purity), light incense, and surround myself with cosy, fluffy blankets, and large pillows. If you like working with water, then get yourself a bowl or cup of filtered or distilled water, and have a fluffy towel nearby. If you have moon water (water charged beneath a full moon), all the better!

2. Allow yourself to soften and settle into this space as you sit in a cross-legged position. If that feels painful in your hips, sit however feels comfortable for you.

3. If you feel drawn to, place your hands to rest lightly on your womb. Breathing in through the nose, allow your breath to travel down through your body, through the belly and into the womb. Exhale through your mouth with a soft sigh. Start to become conscious of your sitting bones – feel them being held by Mother Earth beneath you. You can picture yourself releasing any tension or stress into the Earth as you exhale.

4. Now, place your hands on your feet. It's important to do this with love – as though you are touching a divine being (which you are!). No focusing on dry skin, or unpainted toenails. Only love. If you like, you can gently massage your feet with oils or lotions, infusing your actions with gratitude. Now, utter some words of admiration and appreciation for your feet. Such as, "Bless my feet. Thank you, feet, for helping me to walk so far, for helping to guide the way. I love and honour my feet."

5. If you feel drawn to, splash your feet with the purifying water. Now, envelope them in warmth from the towel.

6. Moving upwards, place your hands on your thighs. Again, massage them, stroke them, and whisper words of love and devotion. "Bless my thighs, my sacred thighs. Thank you for supporting me, for holding me when I most needed it. I love and honour my thighs."

7. Next, gently place your hands over your womb. Spend some time here. Breathe into your womb, stroke and nourish it, and infuse it with love. "Bless my divine womb. My place of power, strength, ancestral wisdom, and magic. I love and honour my sacred womb."

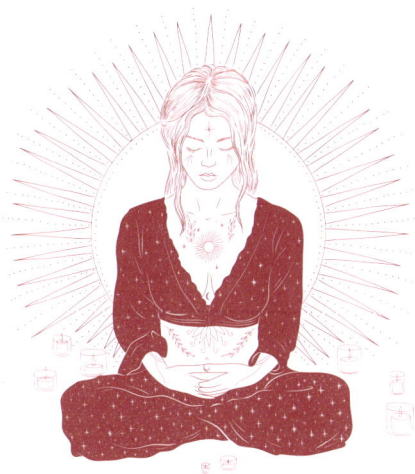

Final Words...

As you cycle and flow through this phase, please remember: health care doesn't need to be prescriptive. Health care *shouldn't* be prescriptive. As you learn more about your body and your cycle, start getting curious about what the different phases mean for *you*.

But, no matter what, remember to come back to this: your body is an altar. Every phase contains magic and super powers. And you, my love, are a walking, talking, radiant Goddess embodied.

8. Continue up the body – tenderly cradling and loving your belly, your breasts, your arms and shoulders, your throat, and your face. Utter words of devotion to yourself. Once you've finished, sit with the energy for a while, or recite a prayer.

9. Finally, if you have one, anoint yourself with a sacred anointing oil. I like to place drops of oil on my third eye, my heart, and my womb. As you do so, you can recite an affirmation that comes to you, such as "I am a divine and radiant Goddess".

10. Stroke and massage your entire body, repeating: "I am a divine and radiant Goddess." Note how you feel when you're finished: how do you feel towards your body? Has your energy shifted in any way? Do you feel heavier, lighter?

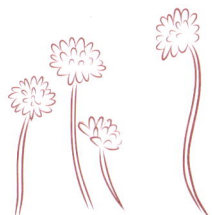

Summer

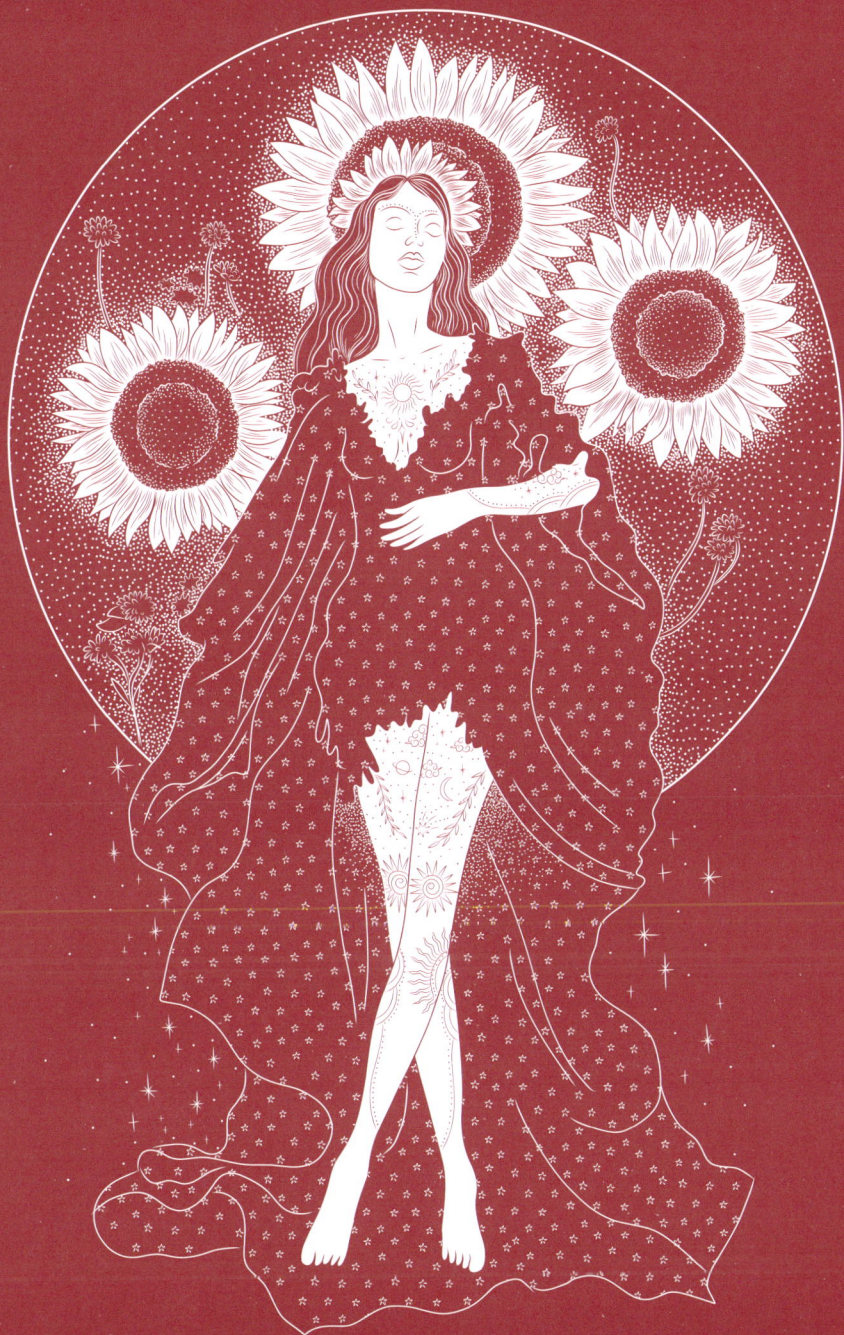

Ovulation, aka Summer

I like to call this phase "Hot Girl Summer". In other words, ovulation – with its sociable, abundant, and fertile energy – is the phase of our cycle that society would most love us to remain in. For many women, this is the phase they feel happiest in. Yet, for others – particularly those who suffer and struggle with conditions such as endometriosis or PCOS, ovulation can be a turbulent time. It definitely isn't always sunshine and rainbows.

Days 13–15 (approx) of your cycle

Archetypes: Lover/mother

Moon phase: Full moon

"She wins who calls herself beautiful and challenges the world to change to truly see her."

Naomi Wolf, *The Beauty Myth*

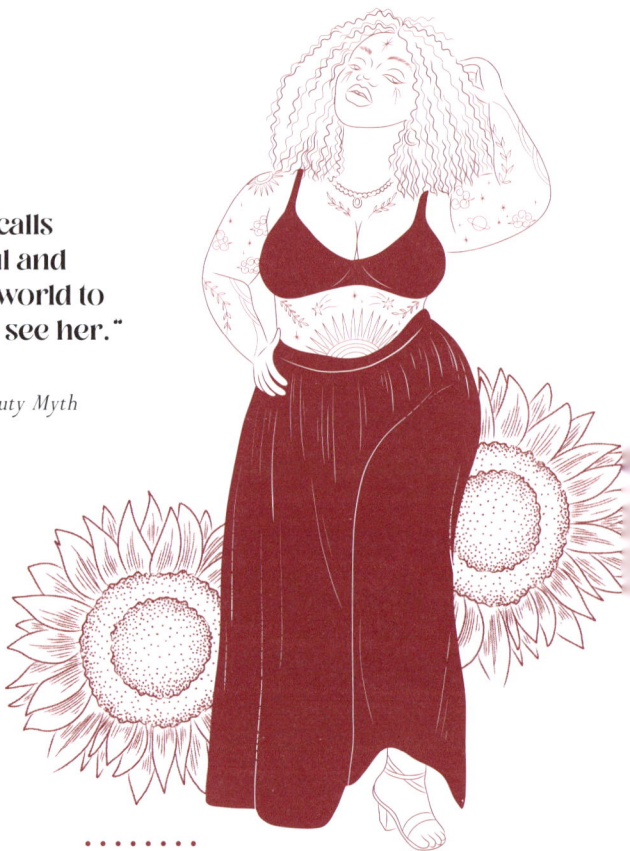

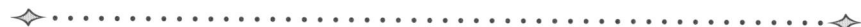

For the most part, though, ovulation comes with more than just a sprinkling of fairy dust. It's where we feel at our most confident and sensual. Our libidos are sky-high, and everything seems like an opportunity. We're full of energy and the nurturing qualities of the Mother. Yet, we also embody the Lover: it's here that we exude magnetism and sensuality. Goddess, you are sexy, and you are utterly alluring. Walk with your head held high, walk with an extra wiggle in your step — and walk in a way that channels those on-screen bombshells. Here, you embody the timeless appeal of Marilyn Monroe, or the super hot Salma Hayek as she hypnotises every single man in the room in *From Dusk Till Dawn*. As you step forwards to embrace your Lover/Mother crown, don't be afraid to be bold, alluring, and confident. Don't be afraid to walk into a room and command all attention. And don't ever be afraid to shine bright.

Around ovulation, oestrogen and testosterone levels reach a gorgeous, juicy peak. This is the main reason why we feel So. Damn. Good. in this phase. If they're in balance, this sassy duo combine to make us feel unstoppable, captivating, confident, and sexy. As we reach this phase of ripeness, a hormone known as luteinising hormone (or LH) surges. This signals for the matured egg to be released, ready for potential fertilisation.

While many of us may think of ovulation as a quick process, it's recently been discovered that it occurs in three phases. In 2024, researchers at the Max Planck Institute became the first to watch the entire ovulation process (observed in mice) under the microscope. I'd encourage you to go online and watch their video. It looks like a mini Big Bang, and shows just how magical our bodies really are — but it's also validating for women who experience pain during this process. The three phases of ovulation were observed to be:

- Follicle expansion, driven by the release of Hyaluronic Acid (HA), causing the follicles to swell.

- Follicle contraction, where smooth muscle cells cause the follicle to contract.

- Follicle rupture, when the egg is released in a mini implosion to begin its journey to meet a potential match in a sperm. Here, the surface of the follicle "bulges outward and eventually ruptures, releasing the follicular fluid, the cumulus cells and, finally, the egg".

You can see why our menstrual cycles need a lot of energy (and fuel!).

Once the egg has been released, the remnants of the follicle which released it start to work their own bit of magic. Without even needing a sprinkling of fairy dust, the follicle transforms into a temporary endocrine gland, known as the corpus luteum. It's this which goes on to pump out progesterone, ready for potential pregnancy, or ready to make our lives (and cycles) much easier in the next phase.

This is why, even if you don't want a baby, ovulation is crucial for our health: without ovulation, we don't get enough progesterone. In fact, I'd go as far as to say that your period isn't the main event of your cycle. Instead, ovulation is.

Ovulation is also associated with better longevity and better health (including healthy bones and lower risk of dementia and heart disease) and lowered inflammation (progesterone is anti-inflammatory). Lara Briden, an author and naturopathic doctor, describes ovulation as "like a monthly deposit into the bank account of long-term health". Of course, ovulation is also associated more directly with good health: we ovulate when our bodies feel safe, healthy, and are thriving.

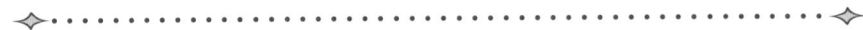

What's Happening Physically?

For those of you who feel vibrant, sassy, and sexy as you ovulate (you don't just feel like a bombshell: you are *The* Bombshell), the actual release of an egg is – sadly – just a 24-hour event. The cycle equivalent of "blink and you'll miss it". Happily though, we get to ride high on that crest of ovulation energy for slightly longer, as our hormones rise and peak in a crescendo. So, if you've ever been curious about what's making you feel so energetic, or so turned on to everything, here's what's going on...

So, how do you know you've ovulated?

Now that we know that ovulation is crucial – whether we want a baby or not – how do you know you've ovulated?

Well, firstly, a period doesn't guarantee ovulation: you can bleed, even if you haven't ovulated. If you find your periods are irregular, it's likely it's not your period that's late – it's your ovulation that was delayed. It's also important to remember that, while ovulation is a one-day event, our bodies are clever (there are even things such as cervical crypts, which store sperm!) and we are fertile for six to seven days.

The easiest way to see where you're at with your cycle is to check your knickers when you go to the bathroom and examine your cervical mucus, or discharge. While some of you may recoil at this, I always encourage women to explore their bodies as intimately as possible. We've been taught that our discharge – just like our blood – is dirty or something which needs cleaning up. Yet, it's crucial for our health. As well as indicating potential fertility, cervical mucus also helps to keep our vaginas clean (our vaginas are self-cleaning – our discharge is part of this), and also helps to transport sperm to the egg (yes – a woman's body is far from passive in the reproductive process, no matter what you've been taught).

So, what are we looking for in our cervical mucus?

Just before you ovulate, you might notice an increase in vaginal discharge. As it increases, it's likely it will be wetter in texture and sticky. As you ovulate, discharge becomes clear and stretchy – it will look like the classic "egg white" between your fingers. Once the Big Event is over, your discharge will slowly become thicker and creamier in colour.

However, this isn't always 100% accurate – sometimes we'll experience that sticky, stretchy discharge even if we haven't ovulated. Another way to check you've ovulated is to track your basal body temperature (BBT) throughout your cycle. This is because our BBT rises slightly after we ovulate (it rises by around 0.2–0.6°C/32–33°F, although this amount can vary with some women) due to the hormone progesterone. If we get pregnant, that temperature rise will be maintained. If we aren't pregnant, it will drop again before our period starts.

There are many apps and products you can use to track ovulation and to log your basal body temperature. However, to use it reliably, I'd advise tracking it for at least three months before using it on its own. It's also important to be aware that some factors, such as sleepless nights, illness and alcohol can impact readings, which is why many doctors do not recommend it as a conception prevention method.

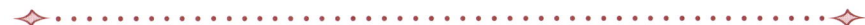

Other ways to track ovulation include monitoring how you feel and even look, and cervical positioning. When we are ovulating, our cervix tends to be higher, and it will become more open and feel softer and wetter. After we ovulate, the cervix can feel firmer and will move lower down.

For some women, particularly those with a sensitive cervix, this can impact your sex life. Positions involving deeper penetration can be painful when our cervix is low and hard. For other women, this can make deep penetration more pleasurable. This is why it's important to educate ourselves, learn about our beautiful bodies, and find what works for us!

Reasons you may not ovulate

If you're not ovulating, what then?

Unfortunately, anovulation (the medical term for not ovulating) can be triggered by all kinds of things. Certain health conditions, including PCOS, endometriosis, and thyroid issues, can all have an impact on ovulation.

A lack of ovulation can also happen when hormones are imbalanced (for example, if we have low oestrogen). It can also occur when our bodies are stressed. This could be caused by extreme exercising, extreme diets, trauma, or emotional stressors. It's also important to understand that women naturally need more body fat than men – while there's no hard and fast rule it's thought that, to ovulate regularly, we need around 22–28% body fat.

If you've just come off the birth control pill, it can also take your body time to adjust and find its rhythm again.

If you're not regularly ovulating, or if you suddenly stop ovulating, see a doctor or medical practitioner for support and guidance.

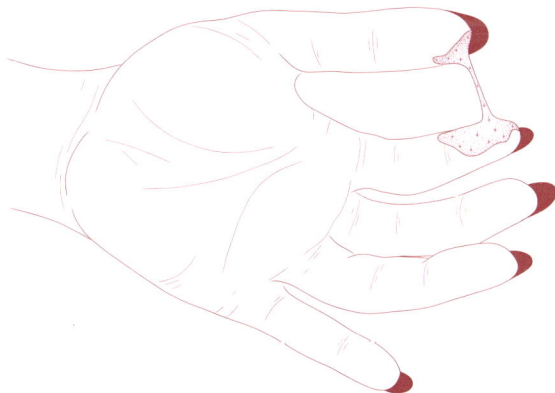

What Else Might You Notice?

Energy

Ever noticed that you feel On Top of the World when you're nearing ovulation?

That peak in oestrogen and testosterone can mean that many of us feel at our most energetic in the ovulation phase. Chances are you feel like Super Woman, and you ooze confidence.

Many mums will also notice they feel more patient and nurturing here. Yet, as a note of caution: as oestrogen's true powers descend on us (or, rather, as oestrogen starts to rise), we can sometimes slip into people-pleaser mode.

This becomes apparent in young girls as they start their periods or begin puberty. I saw it in myself: I was feisty and fiery as a young girl. I spoke my own mind, howled at injustices, and would rage and roar at the world. Yet, as oestrogen starts to rise, this grit and fire and determination can become dampened. Biologically, we become more nurturing, more attentive, more socially pleasing. And, while this is essential for survival – we need those nurturing qualities – beware of people who may be over-stepping your boundaries, or those of any young women in your family or social circle.

Try to become more aware of how people make you feel in this phase. What are you brushing off that you wouldn't usually ignore? What are your instincts telling you? Don't let oestrogen make you forget your own boundaries.

You get some va-va-voom

For many women, ovulation is where we come to understand that we are Goddess Embodied. Even our hips sway with the knowledge that we are total and utter Queens.

You may also notice, when you apply your make-up, that your face looks slightly different, and your skin keeps its radiant, fresh glow. As we ovulate, even our faces can look a little different, softening slightly and very subtly – nature's very own way of making us look more attractive to a potential mate. Studies back this up. Both men and women have been found to judge photographs of ovulating women as "more attractive", while psychologist Geoffrey Miller's infamous lap dancing study found that dancers were likely to be tipped more while they were ovulating.

Sense of smell

One of the surest signs I'm approaching ovulation is that my sense of smell goes into overdrive. I'll walk into a room and instantly notice the slightest whiff of sweat, or the gentlest hint of decay in the fruit bowl. It's not just one of my own quirks, either! Studies have shown that a woman's olfactory abilities (in other words: your sense of smell) can sharpen here.

In particular, studies show that women who aren't on the pill are especially sensitive to male hormones and the smell of musk. While no one knows for sure, it's likely that these changes are evolutionary to help us identify the perfect mate.

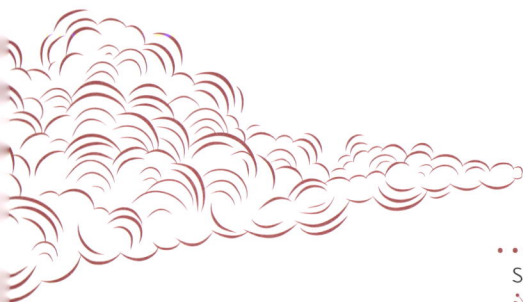

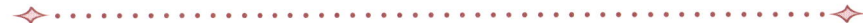

Libido

Find yourself with an extra spark and a twinkle in your eye? You're not alone!

Lots of women find that their libido peaks just before ovulation, and they'll feel hornier and more ready for sex. This is again triggered by a surge in hormones, but it's worth pointing out that it can also be influenced by the sheer fact that we simply feel like Sex Goddesses here.

In fact, I know many a woman who would gladly strut their stuff down the high street in their sexiest bra and knickers in this phase – and then quickly revert back to baggy joggers and slouchy sweatshirts as they near their periods!

If your libido is non-existent or earth-shatteringly low, it could be a sign of hormonal imbalances (such as high or low oestrogen or low testosterone). However, a low libido doesn't always mean that our hormones are awry.

As women, our brains are actually our most important sexual organ. This means that our libido can vanish at the slightest hint of stress, pain, frustration (note to all partners: we won't want sex if you're neglecting your share of chores!), or trauma. Our body image also plays a huge role in our appetite for sex, so please tread gently and with love and compassion if you're lamenting your low libido.

Which leads me onto our first exercise of summer...

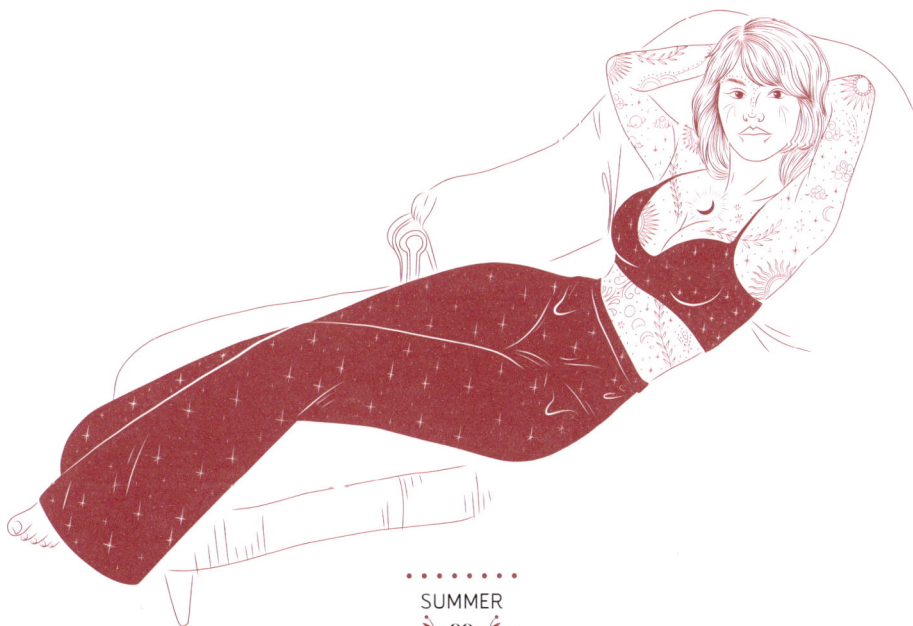

Vulva Gazing

✦ • ✦

While this exercise may be uncomfortable for some, it can be a powerful practice to help us appreciate and honour our gorgeous female form.

It's heavily inspired by Yoni Puja, a sacred Tantric ritual. As you may already know, *yoni* is Sanskrit for our sacred anatomy (it translates as "womb" or "sacred space"), while the word *puja* means "the act of worship". In other words, the Yoni Puja is a beautiful, tantric ritual where the vulva and vagina are admired and worshipped.

1. Create a safe and sacred space for yourself. Your space should be warm and cosy, and it should feel quiet and secluded. You might like to surround yourself with blankets and cushions, burn incense and play relaxing music, but the important thing is: create somewhere where you can relax, and feel completely safe.

2. Consider how you feel about your yoni. What thoughts come to mind when you think of it? What words do you associate with it? Do you feel proud of your yoni, or ashamed and embarrassed? If you feel shame, where might this stem from? Try to attach no judgement to this, just get curious.

3. Now, I'd like you to take a handheld mirror and gaze at your yoni. Spend time here: note the colours, which might range from deep terracotta to the darkest maroon, blush, or ochre. Note the shapes, the patterns, and whether there are any intricate, origami-like folds. Is your clitoris proudly on show, or is it a delicate pearl tucked away? Remember that every vulva is as uniquely beautiful as a snowflake.

4. If you'd like to, and if it feels comfortable and safe to do so, slowly part your lips to unveil the vaginal opening. If you want to continue, you could try gentle vaginal massage, or cupping yourself. It doesn't have to be sexual – the touch can simply be loving, or even curious. You could also do this a second time when you are aroused and see what changes (for example, if your yoni changes in colour, or if it swells and engorges).

5. If you feel drawn to do so, utter words of affirmation or love to your yoni. Tell her that she's beautiful and cherished. Thank her for the wisdom she holds, for the feminine power and magic she helps you to keep safe.

6. Now, close the practice and ceremony. Without any judgement – just loving curiosity – note how you feel. If you feel called to do so, journal about your experience.

A Side Note...

A loving side note for the women who find ovulation to be Inner Hell, with symptoms including:

· Mittelschmerz (aka ovulation pain, which occurs as cramping as the egg is released)

· Bloating or nausea

· Hayfever or allergy-like symptoms

For some women, issues at ovulation can point to PCOS or endometriosis. We've already looked at endometriosis, but PCOS symptoms can look like:

· Missing or irregular periods

· Very light or heavy periods

· Cysts on the ovaries

· Stubborn body weight

· Acne or particularly oily skin

· Facial hair (hirsutism)

· Male-pattern baldness, or thinning hair

· Difficulty getting pregnant

There are different forms of PCOS (and it's important to note, you don't have to have multiple ovarian cysts to be diagnosed with it), but I'd suggest speaking to a doctor if you feel you may be struggling.

As with many symptoms of women's health, ovulation pain isn't widely researched or understood. However, it's thought that symptoms can be triggered by high levels of LH and inflammatory prostaglandins, which trigger muscle contractions. In this case, some women find an improvement in ovulation pain by lowering overall inflammation – avoiding inflammatory foods (such as seed oils, alcohol, and trans fats), supporting your nervous system, and giving your body plenty of love.

For some ideas on how to do this, flick to the Hormone 101 chapter. You can also make the following soothing Golden Milk, which is a great alternative to coffee, as caffeine in particular can worsen symptoms for some women.

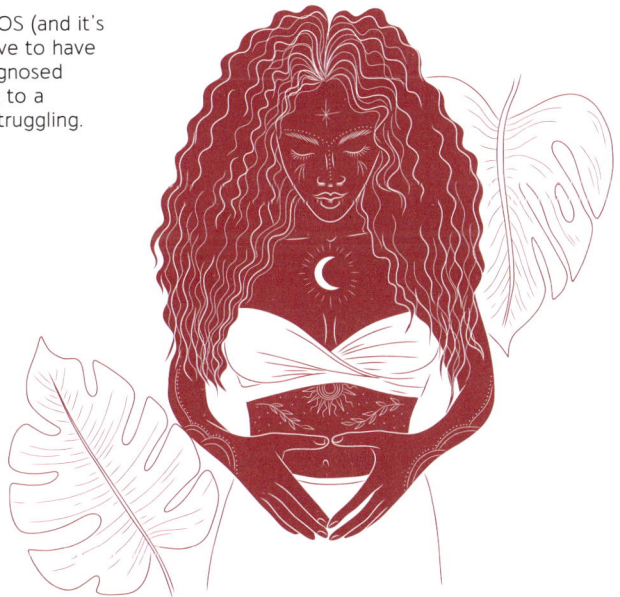

Make a
Golden Milk

◆ • • • • • • • • • • • • • • • • • • • ◆

This delicious, sunny drink contains some of my favourite anti-inflammatory ingredients, such as vibrant turmeric and ginger, which has been proven to ease pain. This warming spice can also reduce any digestive symptoms you may experience, including nausea and bloating.

However, you don't have to struggle with ovulation issues to enjoy this drink! You can also sip and enjoy it at any point in your cycle.

Ingredients:

240ml (8½oz) milk of choice (if using nut milk, try to avoid ones with inflammatory ingredients, such as gums or vegetable oils)

½ tsp ground turmeric

¼–½ tsp ground cinnamon

¼ tsp ground ginger

½ tsp vanilla extract

Pinch of black pepper (this enhances the absorption of the good stuff found in turmeric)

Optional: 1–2 tsp honey or sweetener of choice, one scoop collagen

Method:

In a small saucepan, warm the milk with the spices, stirring often. Stir in the honey, if using, then pour into mugs and enjoy. If using the collagen, pop in a blender and whizz until smooth and frothy.

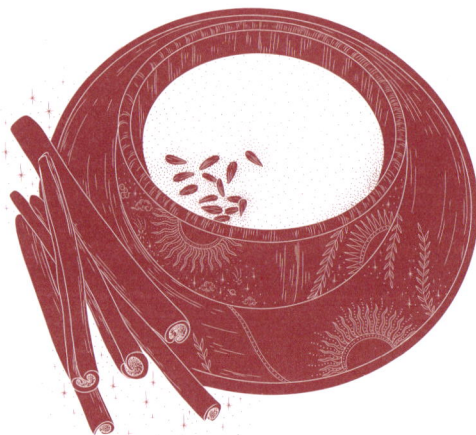

Ovulation and Histamine Intolerance

If you struggle with bloating, headaches, anxiety or allergy-like symptoms at ovulation, this can also point to histamine intolerance.

Without getting too scientific, when oestrogen levels rise, histamine levels also go up. For this reason, women with histamine issues may also experience symptoms before their periods, particularly if progesterone levels are low. This may also be the case for women who struggle with so-called period flu.

Histamines are released by mast cells in response to allergens, which can then cause hayfever-like symptoms, such as sneezing, itchy eyes, and a runny nose, as well as diarrhoea, bloating, headaches, skin issues, or nausea. Oestrogen can also affect diamine oxidase (DAO), which is an enzyme which helps your body to break down histamines.

In a double whammy, high histamines can then lead to *more* circulating oestrogen, which then creates *more* histamine – a vicious circle of the worst kind!

If this sounds familiar, here are a few things to try:

· Support healthy ovulation and lower your stress levels so that you benefit from progesterone. This hormone leads to DAO production.

· Support your gut (flick to the Hormone 101 chapter for ideas on how to do this) to further support DAO levels.

· Help your body to eliminate excess oestrogen by enjoying fibre-rich foods and cruciferous vegetables.

· Consider supplementing with quercetin, magnesium, DAO, and vitamin B6. Consult a trained professional if you're unsure. You can also enjoy plenty of nettle tea.

· Reduce or eliminate histamine-rich foods, such as avocado, spinach, walnuts, aged cheese, smoked fish, vinegar, bone broth, and chocolate.

However, since a low-histamine diet can be very limiting, I wouldn't advise this long term. Instead, work alongside a professional, such as a nutritionist, to try and find the root cause of your histamine issues.

Many women who experience issues at ovulation – such as pain, mood changes, and more – may also want to explore any possible emotional root causes of these symptoms. For example, ovulation problems may be related to times where you aren't birthing your true potential or creating magic (the ovaries are related to creativity), or perhaps you're craving more connection.

On the flip side, some women also struggle with allowing themselves to be seen in all their glory, and want to remain invisible. This can occur for many reasons (some women simply aren't comfortable with outwards energy), but we live in a society that encourages us to blend in and not to stand out.

There are also many women who become overwhelmed by the fizzing, bubbling surge that comes with the crescendo of ovulation energy. If your brain is already over loaded or over active, the addition of peaking oestrogen and testosterone may feel intense. I include myself here: I find that this energy can actually feel too much, particularly when my brain is already whirring with ideas! It's important to remember that, if you don't thrive during ovulation, you are far from alone.

How to Support Your Body

Skin

While your skin is radiant, make the most of that dewy glow, and give your skin a chance to breathe by easing back on make-up.

Be aware that while most women will experience their clearest, brightest skin around ovulation, if your skin breaks out: you're not alone. For some women (for many years, that "some women" included me), a mid-cycle surge in testosterone can cause a rise in sebum, an oily substance in the skin. This is particularly common in women with androgen-related PCOS. We need sebum to help maintain our skin's moisture levels, but too much of anything is often a bad thing. Too much sebum? You'll likely experience blocked pores and acne, especially if there's inflammation in the body.

Treating acne is multi-layered, and there's no "one size fits all" solution as there are multiple causes and underlying issues that can lead to acne. However, my acne – and acne in my clients – has been transformed by introducing lymphatic massage (my favourite guide is *The Book of Lymph* by Lisa Levitt Gainsley, which has simple-to-follow sequences) and by adding a good quality zinc supplement and electrolyte drops to your diet.

Many women will also benefit from using niacinamide-based skincare, as well as balancing blood sugars and introducing purifying face masks, with ingredients such as tea tree or honey. If acne is caused by high androgens, then sipping spearmint tea can also help to bring things into harmony and balance. You'll also want to support your liver and gut (flick to Hormone 101 for more).

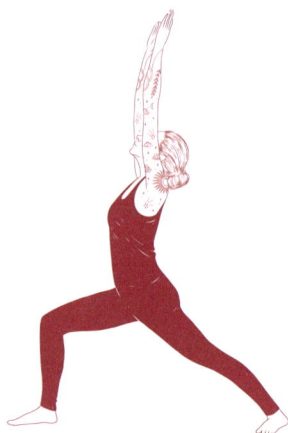

Warrior One

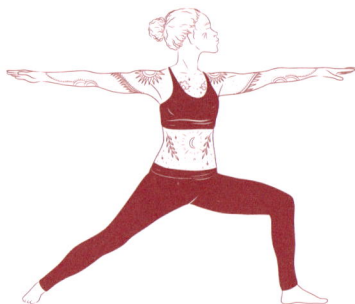

Warrior Two

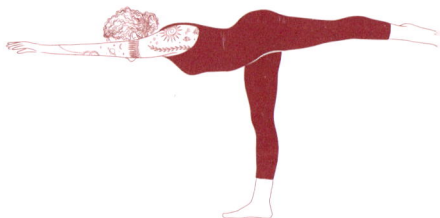

Warrior Three

Yoga for
Summer Heat

✧ • ✧

Want to push yourself but don't fancy lifting weights or trying your hand at conventional cardio? My dear friend Sam Isaacs, whom we met in the Winter chapter, has invited us all to enjoy an Ashtanga yoga practice to help us to unwrap the potency of our summer fire.

This flow of poses allows you to move rhythmically with the breath from one posture to the next, creating heat and *agni* ("fire" in Sanskrit) in the body and unlocking your power. You can give it a go at home, without needing to book into a class, and without needing to follow step-by-step instructions! The intensity of this Ashtanga flow – the heat, power, and energy created in more dynamic practices – will make you feel charged and alive, like the powerful goddess you are.

1. Want to embrace this potency? Nothing invokes power quite like the warrior postures – just make sure you balance out both right and left sides when you do them.

2. Reach your arms tall towards the heavens in Warrior One. Your legs will be in a high lunge position, but with your back heel down and toes angled out to the side.

3. Now, try moving into Warrior Two, with arms reaching wide and stretching out to either side of the body. Here, bend the front knee – toes pointing forwards – and keep the back leg straight behind you, feet angled to the side. Direct your gaze in the direction of the bent knee, hips open and out-stretched.

4. Try focusing your balance on one leg in Warrior Three. With hands outstretched in front of you, or in prayer position at the heart centre, lean forwards, rooting your weight on one foot and raising the back leg.

5. Breathe steadily and assuredly as you hold these intense poses, feet rooted firmly on the ground. You are standing in your power, you are supported, and in knowing that you are even stronger.

6. Using an oil blend in Savasana (the final resting yoga pose, used at the end of sessions) either in a diffuser, or diluted in a carrier oil and applied to pulse points or the third eye, can make an already electric yoga practice feel even more enlivening. Jasmine is the ultimate flower of summer – the small and delicate white flowers are intoxicating and deeply sensual. Chamomile roman is much lighter in its fragrance, yet this plant also holds the power of awakening. It brings a softness and soothing aspect to the summer, which is also true of lavender. A blend can't be complete without a nod to citrus. For summer, grapefruit, sweet orange, and bergamot are queens. They invigorate our soul and make us want to dance in the evening sun – freely, without caution, and uninhibited.

Exercise

This is the time to stretch yourself! Strive for those personal bests. Push yourself to lift heavier weights. Enjoy a new exercise class, or let the sweat drip down as you sprint faster and harder than ever before.

As energy levels peak, you'll likely be able to embrace more intensity, so ramp it up! However, as a word of caution: some studies have shown that women may be more injury-prone at ovulation. Tread carefully, and do some extra warm-ups and stretches to try and avoid hurting yourself!

Food

You may still notice that your appetite is diminished in this phase. This is considered a phase with lots of internal heat in the body. To balance this, many women benefit from enjoying lighter, fresher foods (such as raw salads, vegetables, and fruits), and hydrating foods such as melon and cucumber. However, if you struggle with bloating, you might want to stick with small portions of well-cooked, or well-steamed, easily digestible veggies instead.

Here, our food focus should also be about helping our bodies to metabolise high levels of oestrogen. In particular, our lovely livers play a crucial role in helping our bodies to eliminate, so be sure to give them plenty of TLC. You can support the liver by eating cooked cruciferous vegetables, such as sprouts, cauliflower and cabbage, or adding in liver-supportive herbs, such as nettle and dandelion, or bitters such as rocket.

You may also remember from the last chapter that our guts play a big part in helping our bodies with high oestrogen levels, so continue to enjoy those gut-supportive foods, and keep up with the anti-inflammatory produce!

Progesterone support

Did you resonate with the symptoms of low progesterone from the Introducing your Hormones chapter? If so, you can support your body by making a few adjustments to your diet for the next few weeks of your cycle. Foods which are rich in vitamin B6, such as potatoes, offal and bananas, can help with progesterone production, as can foods high in vitamin C, such as broccoli, red peppers and berries. You may also benefit by increasing your intake of zinc, found in pumpkin seeds and chickpeas, throughout your cycle, as well as magnesium.

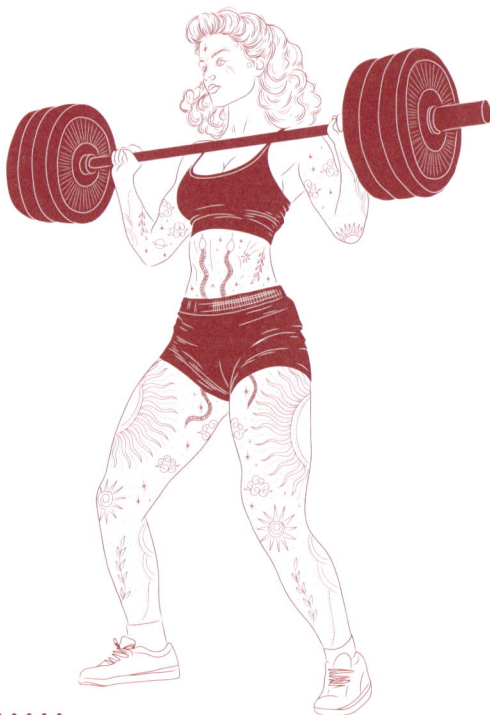

What's Happening Emotionally?

Push yourself and reach for the stars! This is where you have confidence in spades, so stand up in boardrooms, do public speaking, ask for a pay rise, or have difficult conversations with (relative) ease. If you want to make your dreams happen (remember those goals you wanted to manifest from your spring phase?), this is where you can really make a start. In short, while your body is riding high on ovulation energy – girl, enjoy it!

Have fun!

As your body reaches a crescendo, it's time to unpin your hair, shake and shimmy those hips, and have fun!

Embrace this sexy, sensual, confident energy – and embrace that inner (and outer) magnetism. Wear your sexiest knickers, even if it's just to do the food shopping. Dance provocatively in front of your mirror – if only to please and pleasure yourself. Go out partying and dancing with your friends, or get up at 3am to wonder and marvel at the skies and the fullness of the moon. Whatever it is, celebrate the fullness and peak abundance by listing three ways you plan on embracing the fertile energy of ovulation.

Socialise

Oestrogen sees us emerge from the menstrual chrysalis as beautiful, social butterflies. When this hormone is high, our extroverted side tends to come out and play. We bubble and fizz and effervesce in social situations. We sparkle in rooms that may be bursting at the seams with other people. We shimmer and shine in situations where we may ordinarily shrink and hide away.

This is the phase where no one puts you in the corner – and heads will turn wherever you walk.

Embrace your more extroverted tendencies by socialising. Book lunch dates with friends, host dinner parties, or find yourself a new class. Similarly, collaborate, do group work, or book into group workout sessions. However, as a gentle word of caution: don't book in anything which you may regret in a week or two, when your introverted luteal phase may kick in hard!

Sexual healing

While our libido is high, summer is the perfect time for tapping into our sexual power – and for using orgasm to help our bodies to heal. In fact, orgasm is one of the most underrated healers when it comes to our female hormones. The problem is, sex is often shrouded in shame, and female orgasm (and pleasure) is often taboo. And yet, it isn't meant to be this way. Sex is meant to be powerful, deeply sacred, and deeply healing. And there are all kinds of benefits to enjoying regular orgasm (which comes far easier to us at ovulation!). In other words, support your body and your health by enjoying plenty of orgasms (whether alone or in a partnership) – and as a result enjoy:

· More feel-good hormones, such as endorphins, dopamine and serotonin. These can enhance self-esteem, boost pleasure, increase motivation, and make us more creative.

· More oxytocin (the love hormone), which can lower cortisol, reduce blood pressure, and build trust and intimacy, and feelings of love.

· Lower stress levels that, in turn, can lead to a healthier immune system, and reduced hormonal issues.

· Less period pain and PMS

· A healthy lymphatic system, which supports healthy detoxification

· A stronger pelvic floor

· Improved sleep

Now, what are you waiting for...?

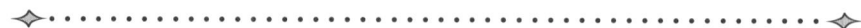

Summer's Super Powers

So, what are your summer super powers? Well, Goddess, there's plenty of magic for you to work with here...

Multi-orgasmic

Most women find they're multi-orgasmic in this phase. This may be because rising hormones can make our clitoris more sensitive, but also because we feel So. Damn. Good. Remember: your brain is a sexual organ.

Take time to explore your sexuality and sensuality. Wear your sexiest clothes – this is where my head-turning, vibrant red bodycon dresses come out to play, or when I slip into low-cut bodysuits and bum-enhancing tight jeans – or experiment with a sexy red lip or sultry eye.

This orgasmic energy can also be used to help you to manifest your dreams – sexual energy is incredibly powerful, and isn't just about how we feel in the moment. When we orgasm, we can achieve heightened consciousness, as well as deep relaxation. Want to give it a go? Before you hit the Big O, think about what it is you want to bring forth into the world. Then, as you orgasm, release and surrender that intention – and let the universe do its work.

Bold and daring

As testosterone and oestrogen soar, our energy becomes more bold and daring, so embrace this fearless energy over the coming days.

Is there something you're dreaming of that you'd like to ask for? Is there a situation that is holding you back? Is there anything you'd like to do that you'd normally be too fearful, too fluttery, or too anxious to try? This is the phase of your cycle where you can – and should – unapologetically Fill. Your. Space. with no fear of rocking the boat.

Stand tall and proud. Wear your crown. Hold your shoulders back and your head high. Supermodel strut as you walk into the room.

Be bold, be daring – and go out and get it!

Communication queen

With the rise in oestrogen, your communication skills peak. You'll appear confident, eloquent and oh-so-knowledgable, and you will sparkle in any social situation. Use that surge of confidence to find ways to use and embrace your voice. What do you feel called to say? What messages do you need to put into the world?

Your super powers include public speaking, presenting, speaking up in meetings or in the boardroom, or trying to get your point across to others. This is the phase of my cycle where I *love* to hold workshops because words tumble out effortlessly, and Everything. Just. Flows.

If this feels too overwhelming, then simply hum or sing – and trust that this positive energy and those vibrations will ripple out into the world.

Similarly, your ability to learn and remember things also peak here. This is because when oestrogen is high, the brain's hippocampus – crucial for storing memories and learning – is thought to grow. So, make the most of this super power, and delve into learning something new, or taking part in a new course.

A Final Word...

As we bid farewell to this season of peak abundance and fertility, many women will feel apprehensive about stepping into the next menstrual phase.

Since our inner autumn can signal PMS, mood swings, and sometimes anxiety and depression, it's difficult to let go of the summer high.

Yet, I ask that you try to keep an open mind about all seasons. While summer may take the glory in our patriarchal world (after all, it's where we can hustle, and it's where we feel sexy, sensual, and super hot), autumn has plenty of its own power...

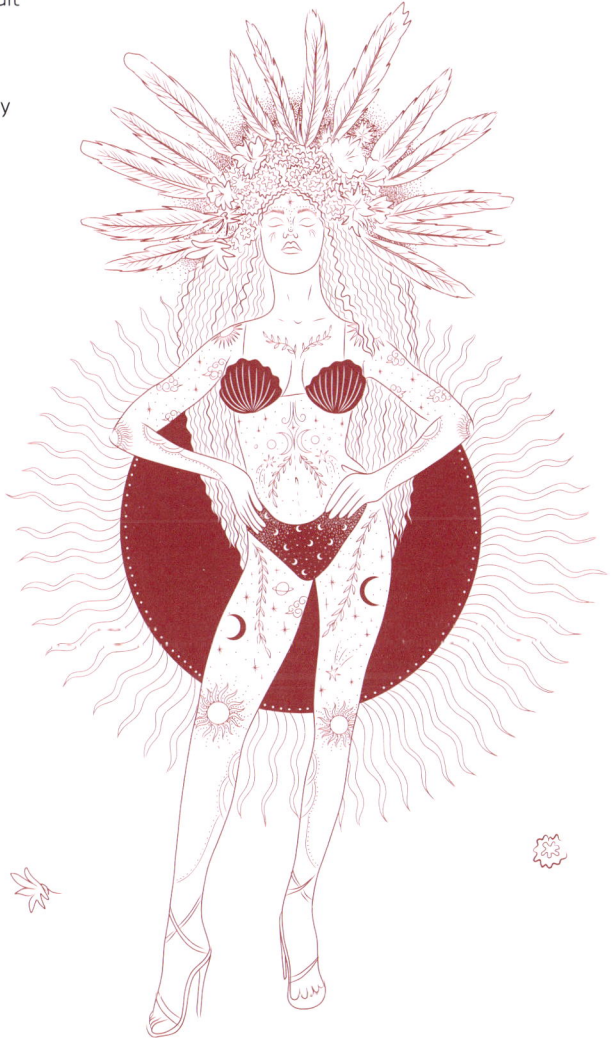

Autumn

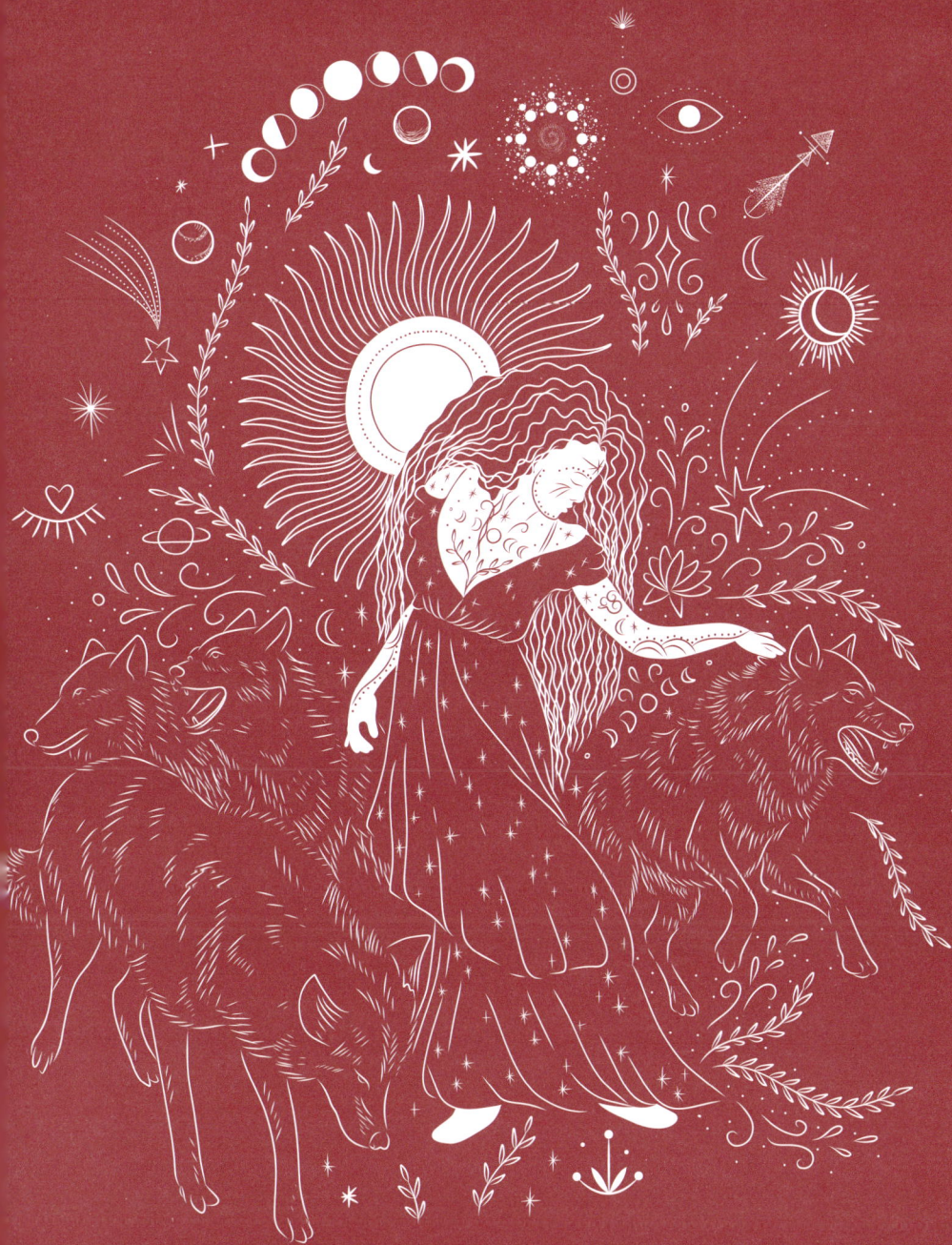

Luteal Phase, aka Autumn

Enter the luteal/autumnal phase – the part of your cycle where you can uncage your wildness, free your inner enchantress, and dance with the wolves. Yet, while the days before we bleed come with an abundance of magic, it's this part of our cycle that we're often demonised for. If summer is the phase society would love us to remain in, autumn is the polar opposite.

Days 16–28 (approx)of your cycle

Archetypes: Wild woman/ enchantress

Moon phase: Waning moon

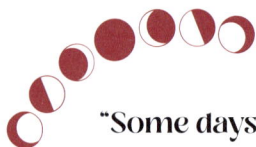

"Some days
I am more wolf
than woman
and I am still learning
how to stop apologising
for my wild."

Nikita Gill, on Instagram

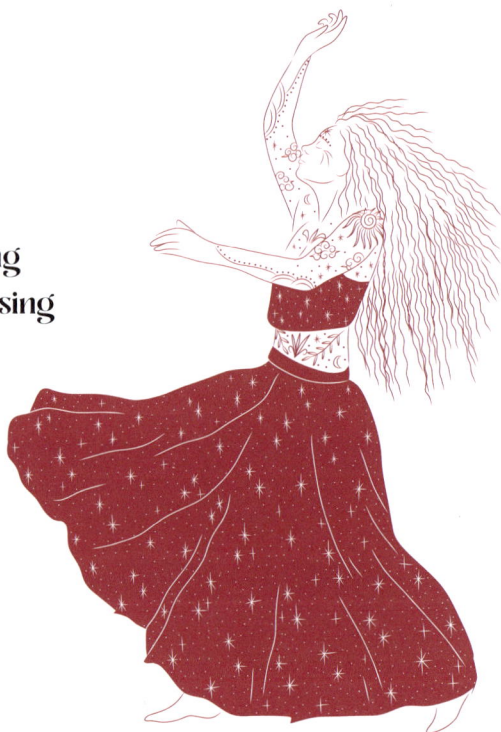

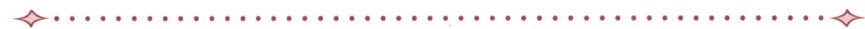

Women who are overwhelmed by their cycles might echo this introductory statement. Perhaps you feel it, too. After all, autumn is the bearer of PMS, breast tenderness, and wild rage and irritability. It's where the lack of education we're given about our beautiful bodies is magnified. If your hormones are out of harmony, autumn can drag you to the depths of hell and back.

For almost the entirety of my cycling years, I'd feel bloated and spotty, angry and raging at the world. My breasts were often so tender, so swollen, that they'd over-spill my bra, and I couldn't hug my boys without yelping in pain. I'd swing between crying at adverts and reality TV, before moving effortlessly into a rage.

Sound familiar?

Yet, after I learned to live in synch with my hormones, the autumn phase (or what I affectionately call my "Wild Woman") has become my favourite. In fact, as I settle down to write this chapter, this is the phase of my cycle I'm currently in – and, believe me, I intended it that way!

While it can feel hot-headed at times, it's here I feel untamed and powerful. It's where I free my Wild Woman so that I can enjoy her inner guidance, wisdom, and clarity. My wildness helps me to understand what isn't working in my life, and what I need to release. After years spent being a Good Girl, of swallowing down my anger and packaging it neatly away, this is now where I drop the mask.

So you see, if you're struggling, there was hope for me, and there's hope for you too. The autumn phase has an abundance of power and magic – and, oh my Goddess, is that magic powerful!

Signs Hormones Aren't Balanced

Unfortunately, wayward hormones make it difficult to harness your inner power.

You may remember from the Meet Your Hormones chapter that there are endless symptoms of PMS and hormonal woes but, if they cause discomfort, affect your day-to-day life, or impact how you see your cycle, you deserve support from your doctor. Classic signs your body is crying out for love include bloating, trouble sleeping, severe mood swings, breast tenderness, night sweats, acne, migraines, or difficulty falling or staying pregnant. These often occur due to chronically high cortisol, an imbalance between progesterone and oestrogen, or when the body is struggling to process excess oestrogen. However, it can also indicate underlying issues, which is why I'd advise professional guidance if needed, particularly if symptoms affect your everyday life or don't disappear. Symptoms can also be more common in perimenopause, or even as early as your late thirties, because progesterone levels naturally decline as we age. You'll find some tricks on how to manage symptoms in this chapter, as well as the next one. But remember: none of it has to be your normal.

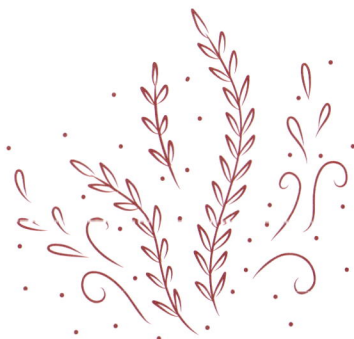

What's Going On?

The luteal phase is the longest of our cycle, but can be split into two halves. When you've just passed ovulation, you're likely still riding high on that wave of energy – the changes as you move into autumn may be subtle after those juicy peaks of oestrogen and testosterone. Then, as you begin to creep ever closer to your period, energy starts to wane, and your Wild Woman takes over. The second week of the luteal phase is what I call "Inner Autumn", and it's where symptoms of PMS can strike.

After ovulation, levels of oestrogen begin to drop. At the same time, lovely, soothing progesterone – produced by the corpus luteum, or what was once the follicle that formed your egg – starts to rise, before taking over the baton. If you aren't pregnant, progesterone peaks about one week into this phase, before dropping once more.

While many women think of progesterone as the star of the luteal show (and, really, it is!) oestrogen also enjoys a resurgence. After initially dropping, it rises once more, before tapering off before your period begins.

So, where do things start to go wrong for so many women?

Unfortunately, because we need the corpus luteum to make progesterone – and because we need to ovulate to form the corpus luteum – things can get sticky for those with anovulatory cycles (the medical term for not ovulating). If you haven't ovulated, you won't experience the Zen-like calm of progesterone, and PMS will quickly become your worst nightmare. If you're struggling with chronically high cortisol, it's also likely that you'll miss out on this soothing hormone. In other words, if your progesterone is flat-lining, or if you're not getting enough, you're in for a turbulent ride. Things also become rocky if your body is struggling to metabolise oestrogen.

What's Happening Physically?

Since we need to address any physical issues before we embrace our autumn power, here's what else you might notice – along with a few tips and tricks to guide you back to harmony.

Bloating

Progesterone is a diuretic, so you may feel more puffy just before your period, which is when levels start to decline. This is common and can continue until the first few days of your bleed. If you're experiencing frequent bloating throughout autumn, it may signal that your body's in "Chronic Stress Mode", or that progesterone levels are low. Energetically, persistent bloating can symbolise swallowed emotions or memories, so it's also worth asking: are there any thoughts I'm suppressing?

Long-term, I'd recommend prioritising restoring gut health, lowering stress, and building progesterone levels. You can find more support on this in the next chapter. However, if you're already scratching your head and wondering what the heck you can do, there are a few things you can try now. Firstly, make sure you're drinking plenty of fluids and eating enough fibre (just don't over-do it – too much of either can also cause issues!), and consider adding electrolyte drops to your morning water for better hydration. Electrolytes can support the skin, brain, mood, and nervous system, and are crucial for overall health.

If you struggle with the Great Bloat, I'd also recommend enjoying potassium-rich foods such as bananas, avocado, and potato, or sipping fennel or mint tea. One of my favourite tricks, though, is to use lymphatic drainage (the amazing book *The Book of Lymph* by Lisa Levitt Gainsley has simple sequences to follow), or abdominal massage, which can restore calm and ease feelings of puffiness almost immediately.

Some women also experience constipation during this phase, which can be caused by *high* progesterone. Digestion can also be impaired by stress, which as we know rises in the luteal phase. Short-term fixes can include magnesium citrate, which eases constipation, or drinking a mixture of chia seeds in water. Sitting in a squat position can also ease constipation. However, long-term it comes down to finding the root cause – and treating it.

Discharge

After ovulation, it's likely you'll see a difference in cervical mucus. After being stretchy and slippery when you're at your most fertile, mucus may become thicker and lose its stretch. It may dry up completely just before you bleed. This is one reason why, if you want to get horizontal with your partner in this phase, you might need lube and you'll definitely want to take things slowly. If you don't fancy sex, don't worry – as hormones change, a dip in desire can be normal, especially if you're struggling with mood shifts. The brain is one of our most important sex organs, so switch the focus to cuddles, and let your partner know.

As an aside, if cervical mucus doesn't change through your cycle, it can indicate hormonal issues, such as low progesterone or low oestrogen. However mucus should never smell fishy, burn, or itch. If this is the case, please visit your doctor.

Blood sugars and stress

Women become more insulin resistant and sensitive to blood sugar changes in the depths of autumn – another reason why you may experience mood swings, fatigue, or anxiety. Studies show that women also experience higher levels of perceived stress (it's thought this is nature's way of helping to sustain healthy pregnancies). What does this mean for you? Frankly, your luteal phase may feel like hell if you don't support your blood sugars – read Hormone 101 for more on that! But, if you're going to do just one thing to ease stress levels and balance your blood sugars now, then start your day with a balanced breakfast. In fact, if you embrace just one thing from this entire book, make it this! A balanced breakfast includes plenty of protein – aim for at least 30g (1oz) – and a serving of healthy fats, such as avocado, as well as nutrient-rich plants. Ideally, you'll eat this within one hour of waking.

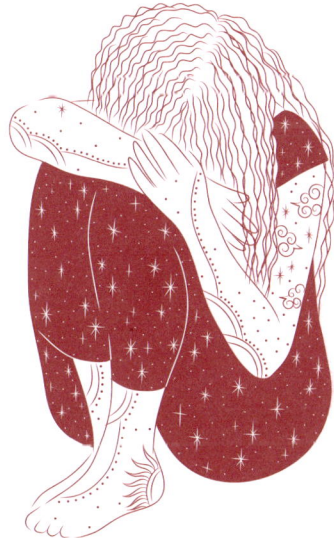

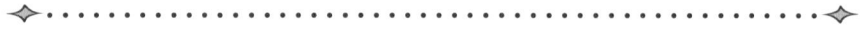

Breast tenderness

One of the most common symptoms of PMS is breast tenderness, which is also triggered by those pesky hormonal fluctuations. This means that you need to address any underlying imbalances to find long-term change. However, many women find relief by ditching caffeine (sorry!) or breast massage, while sore boobs are also linked to low iodine levels. You can try increasing your intake by eating sea moss or organic seaweed sprinkled over some meals, although I'd advise speaking to a nutritional therapist about dosage first. I was able to transform my own breast health by ditching chemical deodorants and wearing a non-wired bra. Underwiring can affect lymphatic drainage, so start experimenting and see how you get on.

Finally, the breasts are related to our heart chakras. If you're experiencing breast tenderness, ask yourself if you could be doing or giving too much without receiving anything in return?

If you experience changes in your breasts, nipples, or notice any lumps, or pain, or discharge, please always consult a doctor.

Skin

Many women – me included! – go from radiant and dewy skin at ovulation to a pre-menstrual oil slick and acne. Others will swap their ovulation glow for dull, dry, and irritated skin. This is again down to hormonal shifts (oestrogen plumps and moisturises), as well higher levels of sebum, which can lead to clogged pores and acne. If your skin is especially dry, it could also indicate low progesterone levels, while acne in this phase can be caused by unchecked oestrogen.

If this sounds familiar, I'd recommend supporting your skin from the inside out. Blood sugar balance is again crucial, as is easing stress and reducing ultra processed foods, and supporting the liver and gut in detoxifying excess hormones. Our skin also benefits from plenty of protein and healthy fats, which work to nourish and moisturise.

I transformed my own skin health and cured my lifelong acne by doing daily lymphatic massage. I also love facial steaming to unclog my pores. When I've moved past ovulation, I use this in combination with soothing, hydrating face masks, or honey and clay masks if I have blemishes.

Some women who experience acne benefit from increasing their zinc and omega-3 fatty acid intake, adding in more minerals (such as electrolyte drops), and quitting dairy produce. Finally, acne can be linked to self-judgement, so tread gently with yourself and give your body (and face) the love and compassion it deserves and needs.

Migraines

I've met many women who are forced to crawl back into bed every month due to pounding, debilitating, pre-menstrual migraines. This is thought to be triggered by dropping oestrogen, which is why some women experience worse symptoms during perimenopause, when oestrogen levels can fluctuate more wildly.

If you're struggling, you may find relief in supplementing with magnesium (this has cured pains entirely for many of my clients) or a B-vitamin complex, both of which can be taken daily. I'd also recommend supporting your blood sugars (I know I sound like a broken record, but they really are *that* important), and keeping electrolytes balanced. Ginger and turmeric are also powerful, natural pain relievers, while peppermint oil can be applied topically with carrier oil to the temples to ease pain.

How to Support the Body Physically

What else does your body need to help you live in harmony with those delicate, female hormones?

Rest

First of all, I'm going to prescribe you rest, rest, and more rest, as your energy levels begin to naturally dip. I know women who have completely cured their PMS through this one change alone. So, see this as your Permission Slip from me: go and run yourself a hot bath, go for a walk in the woods, or curl up with a book.

I know that society doesn't make it easy for us, and I know that you might feel guilty for taking time out. Yet, is it really worth the compromise of frazzled hormones, or feeling on edge and burned out? Didn't think so...

With that in mind, I'd like you to list three gentle ways you can enjoy this rest – every day, if you can. Writing them down is your commitment to yourself and to your sacred body.

Prioritise sleep

If you're below a certain age, getting an early night might seem dull and really unsexy (although, I can't imagine anything more tempting). Yet, sleep is crucial for our health and hormones – and it's especially important in the autumn phase – so bite the bullet and aim to hit the sack an hour earlier.

If you struggle with dropping off when you're in the depths of autumn, especially if this is accompanied by a racing mind, it can suggest low progesterone (remember, this hormone helps you to unwind), and the tips in the Hormone 101 chapter may help. Sleep can also be affected in this phase due to progesterone causing our body temperature to rise. If you find this is the case, having a hot shower or bath before bedtime can help. You might also want to switch to cooling, linen bed clothes and sheets.

Working out

When it comes to exercise, it's important to listen to your body's own cues and energy levels. As you approach autumn, you might still be riding high on crests of ovulation energy, so tune in and keep enjoying intense workouts if you fancy.

However, I'd encourage you to start dialling down the intensity as energy begins to wane. Low-impact workouts – such as swimming, walking or pilates – are especially great in this phase, as is yoga, which can help to release tension. Certain poses – such as lying with your legs against the wall (see the Winter chapter) – can help if you struggle with water retention or overwhelm.

Again, tune into your own needs, and experiment with what works for you! If your body wants more, then go for it. Similarly, if your body is crying out for you to rest... hit snooze on your alarm, and let yourself sleep in!

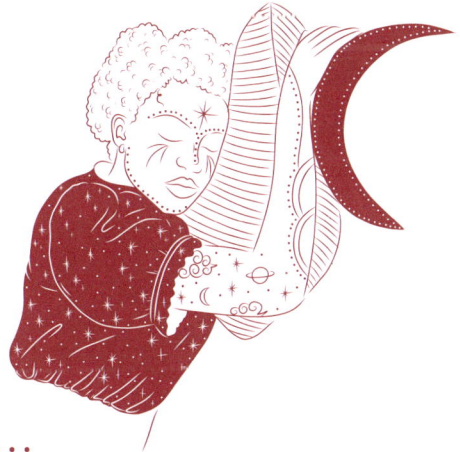

Food

Nutrition will forever be one of my favourite medicines – but never more so than when I reach inner autumn.

As you now know, our bodies are more sensitive to stress and blood sugar changes in autumn. This means it's crucial to eat three, balanced meals a day – no skipping meals or fasting, which will signal danger and send your body spinning into stress mode. Flick to Hormone 101 for more on how to support your blood sugars naturally.

If you tend to feel slightly hungrier in your autumn, this is also normal – our metabolic rate can rise, so let yourself eat a bit more. Studies can't quite agree on how much more we need, but it may be 8–15% more calories. The important message is: listen to and trust your body. If you're hungry, don't feel guilty. Go forth and devour that bar of (dark) chocolate – and no skipping meals!

Here's what else to load your plate with:

Magnesium-rich foods

Magnesium-rich foods can be helpful since this mineral can ease symptoms of PMS, support mood and blood sugar levels, lower inflammation, and reduce pain or tenderness. I advise most women (myself included) to take a good quality supplement throughout the cycle, but magnesium-rich foods to add to meals include dark, leafy greens and cacao.

Embrace the carbs

Fellow carb lovers can rejoice because this is *the* phase of your cycle to enjoy them in! High-carb and high-fibre foods, such as brown rice and quinoa, not only support our thyroid, but they also sustain energy levels and healthy digestion. Progesterone also thrives on glucose, while carbs can even encourage the production of the "happy hormone" serotonin, which tends to nosedive in the luteal phase. Since our blood sugars are more sensitive here, you might like to dress carbs with protein and healthy fats to avoid any spikes or crashes.

Cruciferous veggies

Love them or loathe them, your body needs plenty of cooked cruciferous vegetables, such as sprouts, broccoli, and cauliflower. Without getting too scientific, these foods help your liver to detoxify excess oestrogen. In other words, they'll help you to enjoy more harmony, and less chaos. They can be especially helpful for women who struggle with breast tenderness.

Consider cacao instead of coffee

Unfortunately for those who adore this precious elixir (waving both of my hands here), coffee can trigger jitters, anxiety, and even lead to symptoms of PMS in women who are sensitive to its effects.

Sadly, I'm among those women. While I'll never quit it completely, I avoid coffee entirely in my luteal phase. This is because it can cause cortisol spikes – and, as you might remember, we're more sensitive to stress at this time.

For this reason, whenever I bridge autumn, I indulge my inner chocoholic and pour myself a soothing mug of ceremonial-grade cacao. Which brings us neatly onto our first autumn recipe...

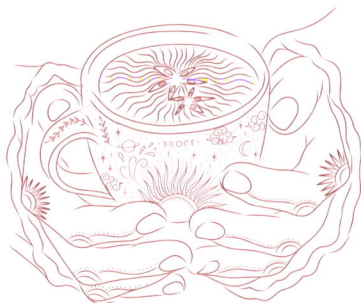

Ceremonial
Cacao Recipe

✧ • ✧

Ceremonial cacao is one of my favourite drinks to sip in place of morning coffee when I'm in my Wild Woman phase. When in its purest form (this means no chocolate laden with chemicals and sugar – sorry!), cacao is gentler on our stress hormones, and can actually support hormone health.

Sipping this liquid velvet can also improve your mood by stimulating the production of happy hormones, while the theobromine found in cacao can gently enhance energy and focus without the coffee comedown. Cacao is also rich in magnesium which, by now, you'll know can work all kinds of wonders.

Yet, the main reason I love cacao is because spiritually it's believed to be a feminine plant. The Mayan goddess of fertility, Ixcacao, is associated with cacao, and the drink can help us to open up the heart space and connect us to spiritual realms.

If you want to soothe away your luteal stressors, then make a ritual out of this drink. Smudge your room with smouldering herbs before making it, say a prayer of gratitude, and set an intention for how you want to feel. You could also write down all the things you wish to release as you approach the end of this menstrual cycle – you can write them in your diary, or symbolically burn the paper (just be careful!).

Here's how I make mine...

Ingredients:

80–120ml (2¾–4oz) water

20–30g (¾–1oz) solid ceremonial cacao, grated

Pinch sea salt

1 tsp maple syrup or coconut sugar (optional)

Optional add-ins: ground ginger (supports digestion and is anti-inflammatory, easing period pain); drop of edible rose oil (rose brings balance to female hormones); ½ tsp vanilla extract (can curb sweet cravings); scoop of collagen

Method:

Gently heat the water and grated cacao in a pan. Stir until the cacao has melted and the mixture is velvety. Whisk in the salt and sweetener if using, as well as any added extras. Pour into a mug, then enjoy!

Note: If you are on some medications (such as certain anti-depressants or blood thinners) or are being treated for conditions such as heart problems, please consult with your doctor before sipping this cacao. If you're unsure, always check with a medical professional first.

What's Happening Emotionally?

Now that you've made yourself a cacao, let's settle down and get to grips with our emotions in this phase. After all, the pre-menstrual weeks can be a bumpy ride. As the hormonal swing starts to take place – and progesterone takes over from oestrogen – our energy draws inwards, becoming introverted and reflective. You may find a sudden urge for time out, and if you're anything like me you may want to become a full-blown hermit. See it as Mother Nature's cue for self-care.

Serotonin – one of our so-called "happy hormones" – can also take a hit in this phase, as can dopamine. This means our capacity for focusing, organising, and even talking can plummet as we reach inner autumn.

Those with ADHD or neurodivergence can be especially sensitive to these changes, but most women will find they feel more tense or on edge, or have an urge to fight fire with fire.

Tools to help mood changes

If you're struggling with overwhelm, breathwork can have a powerful impact on how you feel. It's something I try to do every single day if I can, but I always pepper it into my days during autumn.

My favourite technique is 4/7/8 breathing, which was developed by Dr Andrew Weil to help patients with anxiety. To try it yourself, sit straight and tall. Roll your shoulders back and down, and allow your body to soften.

Breathing in through your nose, inhale for a count of four. Hold the breath for seven counts (or as long as possible), before exhaling for eight. Repeat. The key lies with making your exhale longer than your inhale, which tells your body you're safe.

You can also care for your mood by supplementing with magnesium glycinate – especially helpful for those who struggle with stress and sleep issues – while L-theanine (found in matcha) can instil calm.

Meanwhile, many women benefit from eating omega-3 fatty acids, which are found in foods such as wild salmon, mackerel, and walnuts. These foods can support brain health and may also ease feelings of depression or anxiety. Vitamin D, the so-called sunshine vitamin (although it's actually a hormone!) is also helpful, so you might like to take it as a supplement from October to March, when we're exposed to less sunlight. Foods that contain vitamin C, vitamin B6, and calcium have also been found to be supportive of pre-menstrual mood changes.

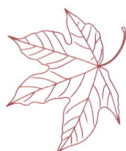

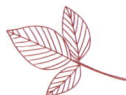

Tread with love...

Given all the emotional changes we're experiencing, we need more love and self-compassion when we're in the depths of autumn. Unfortunately, many women (and I count myself here!) will also feel a strong urge to stand in front of the mirror and pick and pull themselves apart.

For this reason, please don't torture yourself further here by hopping on the scales (I wouldn't recommend that anyway, but that's another story), or trying on new clothes or outfits – especially swimwear. Instead, find yourself some loving words of affirmation to have to hand (my favourite is "I am a radiant, sensual goddess"), indulge in plenty of self-care, and make sure all the outfits that make you feel like the goddess you are are hanging at the front of your wardrobe.

Finally, don't forget the power of a good hug! If you're feeling frazzled, hugs are one of the quickest ways to lower your cortisol. If you don't feel like hugging a person, hugging a pet or even a tree will do.

PMDD

If your emotions are unbearable or feel uncontrollable, it's possible that you have pre-menstrual dysphoric disorder (PMDD). It's thought that women who experience it are particularly sensitive to the luteal phase's hormonal fluctuations, but the causes can be multi-layered. Women who have ADHD or autism are also more likely to experience PMDD.

Symptoms include:

· Frequent low mood or tearfulness

· Feelings of overwhelm or hopelessness

· Suicidal thoughts

· Extreme mood swings

· Lack of interest in things you once enjoyed

· Insomnia

· Feeling extremely tired

· Issues concentrating

· Anxiety

· Persistent anger

I cannot stress enough: if you resonate with any of these symptoms, please contact a doctor or a professional whom you trust. If you need help now and are in the UK, you can call the Samaritans on 116 123. If you're elsewhere in the world, please call a local mental health service. You never have to suffer alone.

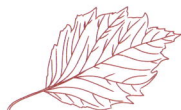

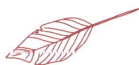

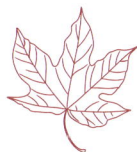

Autumn's Super Powers

While emotional and physical difficulties in the luteal phase are entangled with our hormones, that's not the full story. In fact, although hormonal issues – such as low progesterone – can heighten mood changes, I'm going to go against the grain here and say that some irritability is normal. And, actually, healthy. While you should never feel out of control, I've come to learn that our anger is often sacred, valid and powerful.

Dancing with our Wild Woman

For me, this is where the true magic of autumn lies. As oestrogen drops, the Wild Woman allows us to see things with more clarity. However, to embrace her and our inner powers, we need to be willing to scratch beneath the surface. We need to dance and get curious with our wildness.

With this in mind, next time you're feeling more irritable, ask yourself:

· Am I angry, or am I expressing the fact that I deserve more?

· Am I hot-headed, or have I been squashing down emotions for the rest of the month?

· Am I irrational, or am I doing too much?

· Am I irritable, or am I being assertive when someone has overstepped boundaries?

I know that it's not always simple. We live in a society that demonises our luteal phase because our emotions can be unpredictable. They can bubble up and erupt, and they can be blunt, spiky, or hazardous. Female anger is not often accepted. For most women, this means that they feel as though something is wrong with them the second they creep away from ovulation. They slip on a mask for half of the month, lest they be cast as "psychos" (as an ex-boyfriend once dubbed me). They package their anger up, hoping it never surfaces again.

The problem? When we suppress our emotions, this can kick-start a spiral of high cortisol in the body. No matter how securely we stash them away, our emotions can never disappear. In fact, they have a funny habit of reappearing in different forms. So, next time you're in the depths of inner autumn, why not dare to dance with your inner Wild Woman? Get curious about what your emotions may be trying to tell you, and harness your power in all its glory and light.

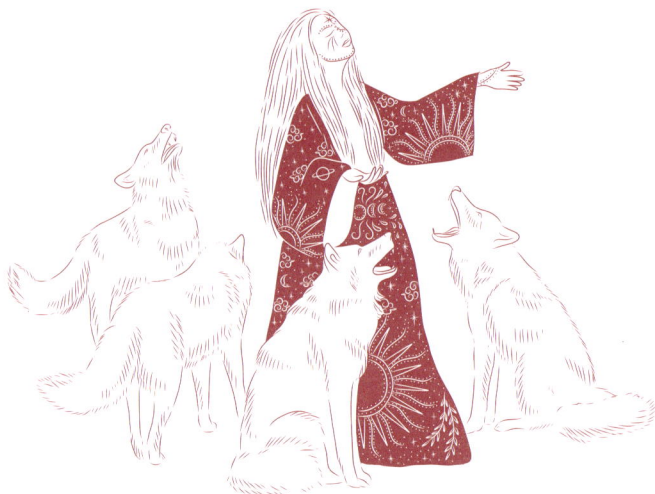

Anger Release
Ritual

✦ • ✦

Whenever I'm feeling tense before my bleed, I hold myself a release ritual to let it out. Shaking (a somatic tool) is a fun and powerful way to release all that's no longer serving me, and is similar to what animals in the wild do when they've experienced danger. Here's how you can try it...

1. Find yourself some music that helps you to channel whatever energy you want to bring forward, or which makes you want to shake, dance, or move. If I'm feeling angry, I like to play Rage Against the Machine. If you really want to embrace this power, you can even dress the part – wear bright red to symbolise power, black to symbolise anger or wildness, or paint eyeliner around your eyes so that you're channelling your inner Wild Woman.

2. Stand with your feet hip-width apart, knees slightly soft. Close your eyes, then slowly start to bounce your legs, before shaking your arms and hands. You can go as gently as you like, or you can ramp up the intensity as you go.

3. If any emotions bubble up, let yourself breathe through them. Shake your entire body, allowing yourself to move in whatever way you feel compelled to. Repeat for as long as needed, before slowing down until you're still. Take a few deep breaths.

4. If needed, get comfy and cosy and sit in stillness afterwards. Reflect on how your body feels, or any sensations that are there.

Tapping into Inner Guidance

So, now you know that our biology and emotions are far from separate. This means that when we experience anxiety or PMS, it isn't just because our hormones are out of whack, or because we're surviving on Ben & Jerry's and desperate to take our swollen, tender bodies and hide out in a dark cave.

Our bodies use symptoms as a language, giving us a glimpse into any underlying emotions that need healing. With this in mind, your premenstrual symptoms or mood changes can hold great power. See them as a monthly report card.

Until I worked on the emotional roots of my symptoms, I was never able to fully heal. Instead, my refusal to rest showed up as heavy, painful bleeds. My lack of self-care – alongside always giving, giving, giving – showed up as breast tenderness. Meanwhile, avoiding my shadows and refusing to work through traumas meant my body grew ovarian cysts.

Believe me, no matter how much your hormones may need love and support, there's often an emotional root to your symptoms. This is echoed in Traditional Chinese Medicine, which acknowledges the emotions we hold within each organ. For instance, our livers – which play an important role in hormone health – are thought to hold anger and resentment, while the kidneys hold stress and fear.

Of course, it takes commitment to harness this wisdom, and it may need us to slow down so that we are able to tap into that inner guidance.

Anything you're struggling with in this phase does not need to simply be dismissed as "hormonal imbalances". These symptoms are your body's way of guiding you back to love, and this is where the next exercise comes in.

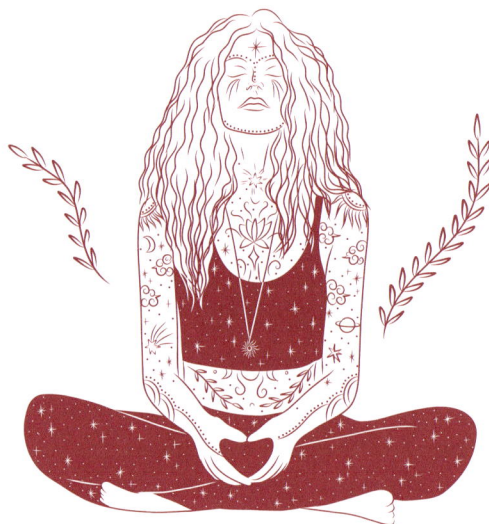

Womb Work
Ritual

✧ • • • • • • • • • • • • • • • • • • • ✧

While diet and lifestyle changes have supported my hormones, nothing has helped my healing more than womb work and daily womb breathing. Using womb work, you can ask yourself the big questions you need answers to, such as: what do you need to release and let go of? What's no longer serving you? What does your body need from you?

This is because many women hold memories and traumas in their pelvic spaces. Our wombs can hold onto sexual trauma, money worries and fears, painful emotions, unbirthed creativity, and dreams unloved and untold.

When our wombs carry emotional and physical baggage, we're more likely to experience dysregulated nervous systems, as well as pain or hormonal woes. We're also more likely to miss out on untapped wisdom, sacred sexuality, and confidence. In short, our wombs hold glimmers of wisdom needed for healing.

I've worked with women who saw chronic hip pain melt away when they started this exercise, and I've worked with others who were able to find the root cause of their hormonal issues – that no doctor had yet been able to guide them towards.

You can practise this simple exercise whenever you have time to yourself, or when you feel called to connect to your body. However, it's especially powerful in your Wild Woman phase. If you like, you can go deeper by asking your womb questions (such as, "What do I need to know right now?", or "What is my body asking me to release?").

1. Sit or lie somewhere quiet, and get comfy and cosy. Let yourself soften and relax, rolling your shoulders back and down and softening your entire body, letting yourself melt into the surface beneath you.

2. Arrange your hands into a downwards triangle (thumbs together, forefingers also pressed together), and lay them over your womb space, just beneath your belly button.

3. Breathe in through your nose, allowing the breath to travel down through the throat and belly, finally filling up your womb. As you exhale, soften and part the lips – this helps to ease tension in the pelvis – and let the breath go with a sigh.

4. If you'd like to, picture the breath as a river, or as liquid, golden light, filling your womb with powerful, healing energy.

5. Repeat for as long as you'd like. Note any feelings you experience as you do this, such as warmth or tingling. If you feel resistance or struggle to connect to your womb, that's also OK. Recognise this without judgement, and try again another time. Thank your womb for this powerful connection, knowing that you can always come back to your body whenever you need guidance or clarity.

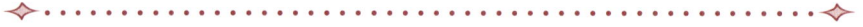

What Other Super Powers Do We Hold?

Cutting through BS

Thanks to our incredible inner Wild Woman, the luteal phase is ideal for first dates. Yes, you might need to pull on your biggest knickers and wear an elasticated waist. Yes, you may not feel your sexiest. Yet, you're also a Walking, Talking Human Lie Detector, and you're far more likely to see through any toxic, manipulative BS.

Dream journal

Have you ever noticed your dreams become more vivid as you creep towards your period? In their book *The Wise Wound*, Penelope Shuttle and Peter Redgrove likened the effects of PMS to sleep deprivation – or, rather, dream deprivation. They say that it's normal in the pre-menstrual phase to experience deep sleep and dreams, and that we can suffer and struggle if we don't.

Our dreams also carry wisdom and guidance, and they can be a powerful way to understand the inner workings of body and mind. To really enjoy your super power of heightened intuition, why not keep a dream journal by your bed? Do your dreams offer up any insights you may need?

Some women may also enjoy using oracle cards or tarot decks here, while others will be drawn to journalling or free writing. Whatever it is you feel called to do, allow yourself to harness your inner wisdom.

Spring cleaning

If you find yourself in nesting mode in the week before your period, you're not alone. In fact, many women will find an urge to Get. Things. Done.

I have ADHD and it's rare (very rare) that I feel drawn to clean. Come into my home and you'll be greeted by a hurricane, with mountains of books (each one started, but never finished), parcels stacked, and sheaths of paperwork that I feel too overwhelmed to flick through.

Yet, this is the phase of my cycle where I feel compelled to tidy, or to dust shadowy corners, sort musty cupboards, clean month-old spinach from the back of the fridge (yuck), and then cleanse the house with a smudge stick.

Many women also enjoy meal prepping here, or ploughing through detail-oriented tasks, such as accounting, reports, and admin. See this as your final super power. It's your body's way of helping you to clean your space and ease stress, so that you can relax and slip into that dreamy energy as soon as you bleed.

Your magic lies in your cycle.

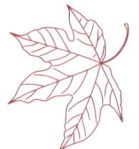

Final Thoughts...

Speaking your truth and unleashing righteous anger isn't PMS. Instead, it's your inner Wild Woman refusing to bow down. She recognises her own worth and her own power – and she will not let you bow down to anyone who doesn't deserve you.

Don't be so quick to dismiss her, and don't allow anyone to make you doubt her and your own righteous anger. Embrace her, and embrace your inner power – and, Goddess, I promise you that your luteal magic won't be far behind.

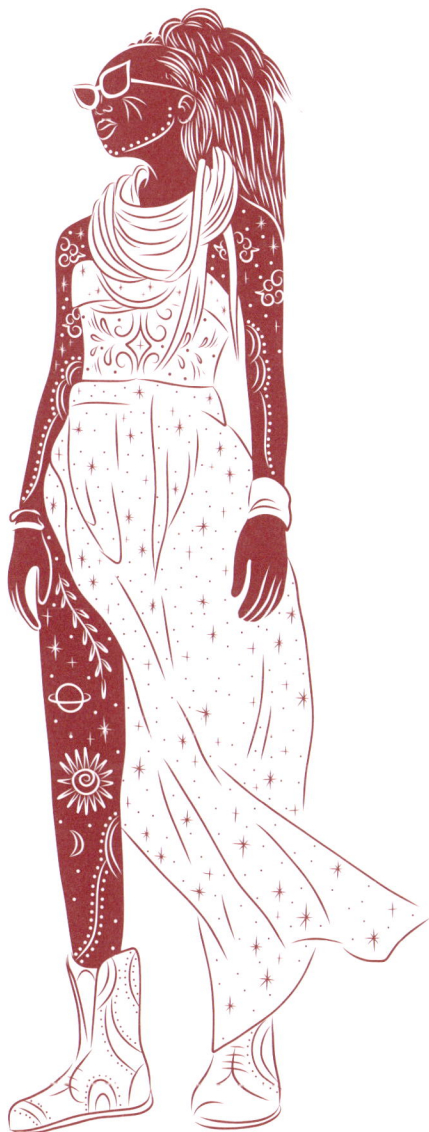

Cycle Tracker

Cycle tracking is a great way to create a record of how your unique cycle looks and feels, and can help you to better understand your own needs. Use this template, or scan the QR code to download a printable copy, and try to fill it in every day.

Monday

Date .... Cycle day .... Moon phase ....

I'm feeling ....

Energy levels are ....My mood is ....

Symptoms I'm experiencing ....

Three ways my body needs support right now ....

....

....

Tuesday

Date .... Cycle day .... Moon phase ....

I'm feeling ....

Energy levels are ....My mood is ....

Symptoms I'm experiencing ....

Three ways my body needs support right now ....

....

....

Wednesday

Date .... Cycle day .... Moon phase ....

I'm feeling ....

Energy levels are ....My mood is ....

Symptoms I'm experiencing ....

Three ways my body needs support right now ....

....

....

Thursday

Date .... Cycle day .... Moon phase ....

I'm feeling ....

Energy levels are ....My mood is ....

Symptoms I'm experiencing ....

Three ways my body needs support right now ....

....

....

Friday

Date .... Cycle day .... Moon phase ....

I'm feeling ....

Energy levels are ....My mood is ....

Symptoms I'm experiencing ....

Three ways my body needs support right now ....

....

....

Saturday

Date .... Cycle day .... Moon phase ....

I'm feeling ....

Energy levels are ....My mood is ....

Symptoms I'm experiencing ....

Three ways my body needs support right now ....

....

....

Sunday

Date .... Cycle day .... Moon phase ....

I'm feeling ....

Energy levels are ....My mood is ....

Symptoms I'm experiencing ....

Three ways my body needs support right now ....

....

....

Hormone 101

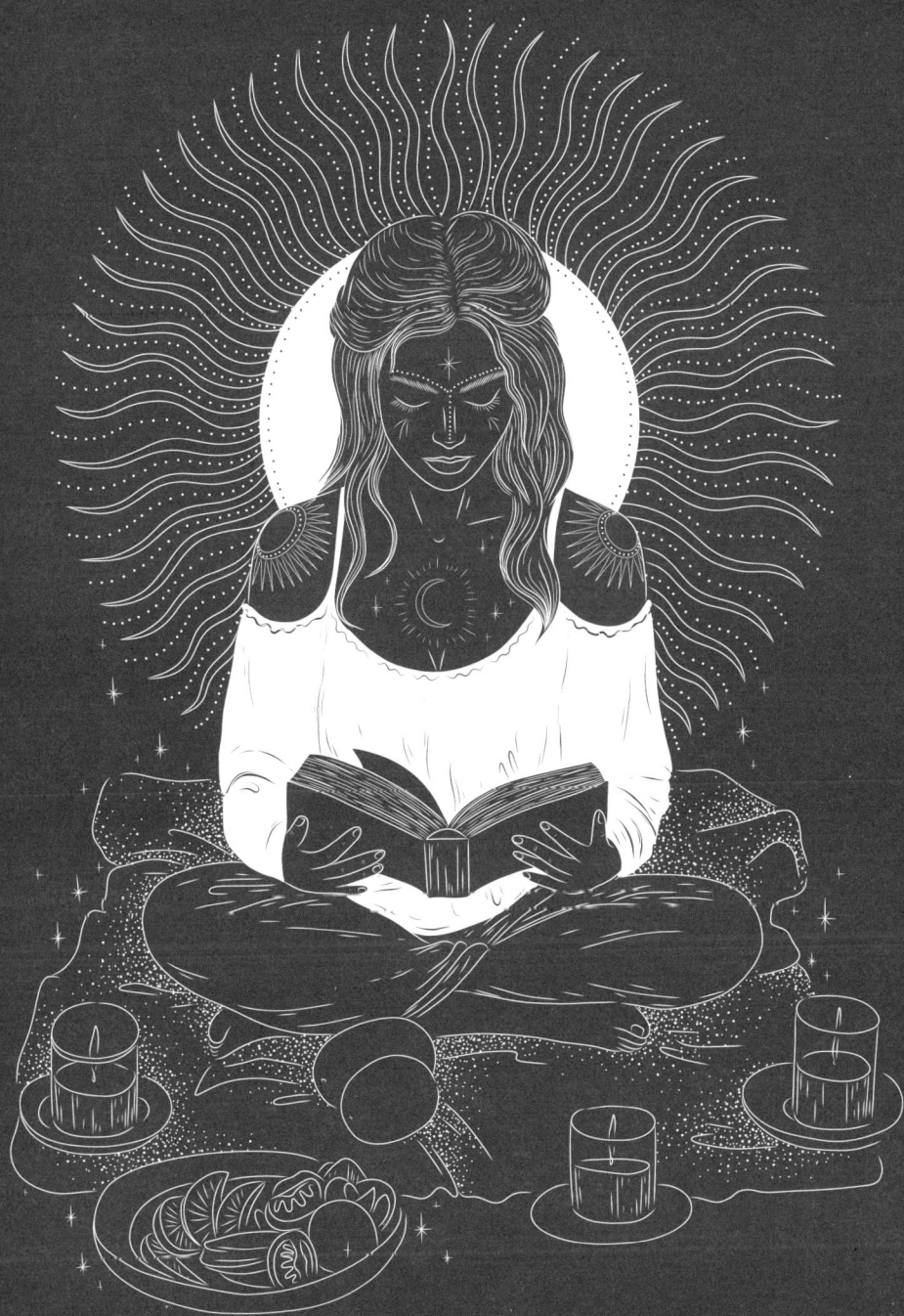

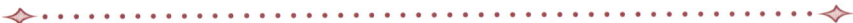

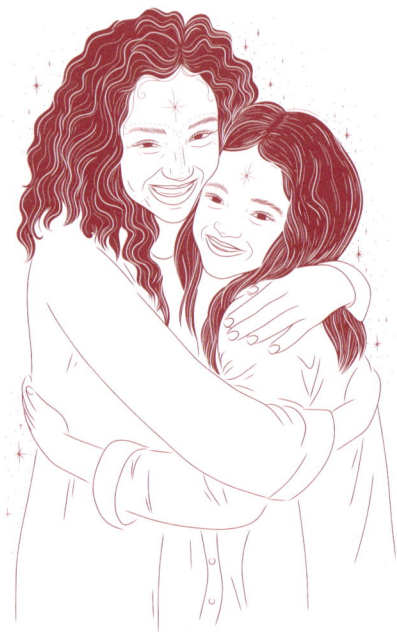

> **"The girl you once were, heal for her.**
>
> **The woman you are now, protect her.**
>
> **The queen you were created to be, fight for her."**

Morgan Richard Olivier,
The Strength That Stays

Thank you for coming this far.

I hope that as you've read, you've had glimmers of wisdom and insights about your health. I hope that you've learned many things about your body, as well as a thing or two about how you can support your menstrual cycle. Perhaps even learn to enjoy it.

Want to learn some more?

This final chapter is what I like to call my "Hormone 101". Alongside cyclical living, the things I will be sharing form my pillars to hormone health. So, pour yourself a ceremonial cacao, snuggle into your favourite blanket, and let's deep dive into some more health-loving practices and rituals for you to try.

Nervous System

If you want to heal your hormones – in fact, if you want to heal anything – you have to give your nervous system some love.

If your body feels safe, you'll thrive. On the flip side, if it doesn't feel safe, then you'll struggle with all manner of things: low energy, poor sleep, PMS, period pain and stubborn weight gain to name a few. Unfortunately, many women are stressed to the max. Stress has also become normalised in this era of chronic productivity – and women are rarely supported through it.

My own health was transformed when I healed the pain I was always running and hiding from. At times, I felt overwhelmed, and I didn't know how to come up for air. And yet, I wouldn't be here if I hadn't worked with a therapist, and I wouldn't be here if I had run from my pain for much longer. If you are carrying emotional pain – or if you struggle with PMDD, anxiety, PTSD, or depression – it might help you (and your hormones) to seek professional support and guidance from someone you trust. It's also crucial to find the root of nervous system dysregulation.

However, in the meantime, here are some of my favourite ways to build safety in the body.

Grounding

Whenever I feel overwhelmed or frazzled, I like to tread my feet into dusty, dry earth, or curl my toes into sweet, damp grass as the rain falls. I walk barefoot through technicolour fields of wildflowers, or paddle in salty, stormy seas. Basically, I like getting my bare feet dirty and onto the Earth.

And when I do? I feel instantly soothed and calmed.

It sounds woo-woo (although, nothing wrong with that – give me *all* the woo), but grounding is rooted in science, and it's all the more important for those of us who spend our days indoors.

Grounding has been shown to support thyroid health, improve sleep, lower inflammation, reduce chronic pain, and support adrenal and hormone health. It can also lower stress and anxiety. So, ditch the shoes, and go and find somewhere to ground yourself and soak up the Earth's electrons.

Breathing

Breath is one of our most powerful healers. Yet, many of us don't breathe optimally, and this can stress the body, trigger panic attacks, cause fatigue, and impact health.

Thankfully, it's easy to start to breathe in a way that supports your health, your nervous system, and your hormones. You can try 4/7/8 breathing, as we learned in the last chapter. Or, you might also like box breathing. To do this, pick a number you feel comfortable with – let's say six, for the purpose of writing – and then inhale for that count. Hold the breath at the top of the inhale for a count of six, then exhale for six, and hold for six before inhaling and starting the cycle again.

However, please be aware that some people who have experienced trauma can feel jittery and anxious when they do controlled breath work exercises. If this is you, please stop and consider seeking support.

Butterfly hug

This is my favourite practice of them all as it feels deeply nourishing and loving.

It's a therapeutic eye movement desensitisation and reprocessing (EMDR) technique that can be used to ground and calm anxiety or overwhelm. To try it, take a deep breath and close your eyes. Cross forearms across your chest, and interlock thumbs to form "butterfly wings". With hands resting gently on your chest, start tapping, alternating hands. Do this for a few minutes, breathing deeply as you tap and picturing clouds drifting across the sky.

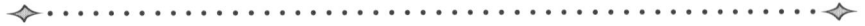

Hug

Don't have time for much else? Have a hug!

Hugs release oxytocin, the "love hormone", and lower cortisol. If you don't have a partner or loved one around, you could try hugging a pet, or even a tree. Other ways to boost oxytocin include orgasm, massage, and gazing into a loved one's eyes. Oxytocin is especially important for women, and is crucial for regulating our hormones and helping us to thrive. In fact, I'd go as far as to say that women need lots of physical connection (which releases oxytocin) to function even nearly at our best.

Singing or humming

Singing or humming is another foolproof way to calm the body. This is because it stimulates the vagus nerve, which plays an important role in calming the body.

Another reason I encourage singing is because our pelvic bowl is intimately connected to the throat and jaw. If you carry tension in your jaw, it's likely that you're also holding tension in the womb or pelvis. This is because our mouth and womb develop together in utero, while our fascia also connects the jaw and pelvis. If you Google the larynx and our womb and fallopian tubes, you'll find they even look similar!

This magic means that singing and humming can both regulate our nervous system, and completely shift the energy in our womb spaces. As a result, singing and humming can be powerfully, deeply healing for women – and the vibrations released when we sing can also help us to put healing energy out into the world for others, too.

Listen to Your Body

The next of my pillars? Tune in and listen to what your own Wild Woman is telling you.

Remember, your body speaks to you in symptoms. Trust in your innate wisdom, listen, and remember: no one will ever know your body better than you do. Also, talk to yourself with love and compassion. Japanese author Masaru Emoto proposed that the molecular structure of water became more beautiful if spoken to with kindness. If it was spoken to with venom or ignored, the water formed patterns that were less intricate. Knowing that our bodies are mostly formed of water, imagine what feeding yourself words of love could do.

Stretching

Women carry many of their traumas and emotional debris in their hips and pelvic bowls. This is partly because our hips are mobilised for quick movement whenever we feel stressed or tense. Tight or shortened psoas muscles (which support hip mobility and connect the torso to the lower body) are also directly linked to period pain, and can play a role in the quality of our breathing and the health of our organs (for example, the psoas acts as a shelf for our digestive organs). For this reason, the health of your psoas is crucial, and many women will benefit from working with a practitioner to ease any tension.

However, as you now know, our wombs are also where we hold all kinds of pain. This means that hormonal issues - or any pain or tension felt in the hips - can occur when we're holding things we need to release. To help your body, you might like to build in a hip stretching routine, or search for suitable online classes (there are lots of free ones on YouTube). Exercises to try include Pigeon pose, low lunges or Goddess squats, or Child's pose for something more gentle. Just tread softly – especially at first – and ask for help if needed.

Other exercises I love for releasing tension include belly dancing, somatic work – which is why I've just finished training in this powerful practice – and shaking it out.

Sleep

I find it hard to write about sleep because, as you now know, I struggled with insomnia for swathes of my adult years. I know only too well how stressful it can be to read how much we need to sleep – and how bad it is for our health when we don't. If you do struggle with sleep, feel free to skim over this section! However, for those of you who want to hear more, here are the tips that have transformed my own sleep:

Support your circadian rhythm

As well as having an infradian rhythm to consider, our body also beats to a circadian rhythm (aka your sleep/wake cycle). When our circadian rhythm is wobbly or scattered, it can become difficult to sleep.

Support your circadian rhythm by waking and going to bed at the same time each day and ensuring you get outside and enjoy plenty of morning light exposure. Other ways to support the circadian rhythm include watching the sun rise and set, and eating regular meals. It's even thought that eating foods that are in season can help to support our internal rhythms.

Avoid caffeine

If you are anything like me, drinking coffee at the wrong time can leave you a jittering, anxious, shaking wreck. If I even dare to sniff coffee after midday, I can guarantee that I'll be staring at the ceiling until the early hours. If you're sensitive to coffee, avoid drinking it in the afternoon wherever you can. Similarly, alcohol can be disruptive to sleep.

Red light therapy

It sounds dramatic, but I'm going to say it anyway: red light therapy has changed my life. Since I started using my red light box morning and night, my sleep has never been better! Red light therapy is less disruptive to our sleep cycles than blue light – and, while more evidence is needed (beyond my anecdotal "it changed my life!"), it's thought to stimulate melatonin, aka the Vampire Hormone (because it's produced at night). Red light therapy may also work by reducing inflammation, supporting thyroid health, and soothing and calming the nervous system.

Swap screens for candles

At the opposite end of the spectrum, we're often bombarded by bright (blue) light via our screens and phones. Unfortunately, this suppresses our sleep hormone and can raise stress hormones, making it difficult to nod off.

If you're struggling with sleep, switch off screens at least one hour before bed. If you feel up for a challenge, you could ditch the screens at night altogether – and even forgo lights! Replacing lights with candles and swapping TV box sets for reading has transformed the sleep of many of my clients. Some women also find their sleep is transformed by sleeping on a grounding sheet, which connects us to the Earth. They can be a little pricey, but they can also be extremely effective!

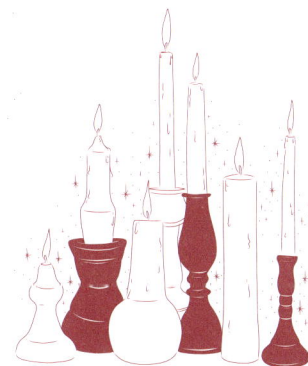

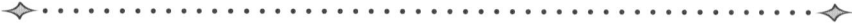

Exercise

After I had my first child, I used exercise to help me cope. I'd push myself to my absolute limit – purple-faced, dripping with sweat – and exercise for hours at a time to help me to process these new feelings and emotions, and all the overwhelming stressors that had suddenly morphed into my life. At first, the exercise worked: I looked great, and I felt energetic and even sexy. Yet, eventually, it stopped working. My body was exhausted and fatigued, I couldn't sleep, and I even started to gain weight. Weight that wouldn't shift, no matter how much more I worked out, or how few calories I ate.

The more I've learned about women's health and hormones, the more I realised I had it all wrong. Pushing my body to its limits every day meant that my body saw exercise as a stressor – and this is why I gained weight.

So, exercise and movement are great! They support our health and our hormones, boost circulation, and add essential muscle and tone to the body. Done right, they can also help us to ease stress. Women especially benefit from weight training, particularly as we move into our perimenopausal years. Weight lifting can help us to build strong and healthy bones, and can also build muscle (which, in turn, helps to prevent weight gain when hormone levels can be swinging wildly).

However, if your body is in overdrive, consider slowing it down – or even resting to allow yourself to replenish. I know this goes against the grain, and I know it seems counter-intuitive. But I promise you: if you are gaining weight and moving more and more, consider that your body may be seeing it as a stressor. The key? We always want to help our bodies to feel safe. Tune into your own energy levels, and move in a way that brings you joy!

Food

I cannot stress this enough: you need to eat enough to fuel your body and your hormones.

I know that this might seem confusing if, like me, you grew up in the era of surviving on ridiculous diets. Yes, restricting yourself to 1,000 calories a day may lead to short-term weight loss, but it will likely cause a cascade of health issues long-term – and you may also end up gaining weight to boot.

It comes down to creating that sense of safety again. Our bodies need food to build healthy hormones, and to signal to our bodies that we aren't in danger. See it like this: when you restrict calories or macronutrients, your body doesn't know that you're dieting and want to feel good in a bikini. Instead, it merely fires off a red alert, thinking you're living in a place with not enough food, or even famine!

Just how much food we need varies from woman to woman, so you might like to consult a nutritionist. However, please do *not* skip meals (not feeling hungry isn't the flex you think it is, and can suggest we're in stress mode).

When it comes to what to eat, I don't have any fresh, exciting nuggets of wisdom to share. Our bodies need plenty of healthy fats and protein, which are the building blocks of our hormones, and we also need complex carbs (think sweet potatoes, ripe fruits, brown rice and quinoa). Please don't fear carbs, or try long-term Keto diets – our thyroid and energy levels need carbs to thrive.

In other words, all the macronutrients matter – don't cut them out!

So, are there any other ingredients you need for your hormones to thrive?

Well, firstly: please try to limit ultra-processed foods wherever possible. This doesn't mean you have to swear off your favourite ice cream or pizza. In fact, please don't – restriction is never healthy, and joy is important for health. Let yourself eat your favourite things!

However, hormones thrive when you limit junk foods and processed oils (such as vegetable oil), instead, eat more whole foods (really, it comes down to that 80/20 rule – 80% of the health-giving stuff and 20% happy treats).

My second tip: try to eat the rainbow! Whether we pile our plates with ripe and juicy tomatoes or strawberries, vibrant leafy greens or plump blueberries, we need to get as much colour into our diets as possible so we get an array of nutrients (and a variety of produce to give our guts some love).

Another important tip is to consider your levels of inflammation. When bodies are angry and inflamed, we're more likely to experience painful periods – and we're also more likely to experience chronic illnesses, and weight gain. Try to include plenty of anti-inflammatory foods in your diet, such as oily fish, turmeric, ginger, berries, and green tea.

Blood sugars

I can't finish this mini section on food without mentioning your blood sugars. I know, I know – I've talked about it before! But, it's crucial. If your blood sugars are haywire, chances are you'll experience all kinds of hormonal issues, as well as anxiety, fatigue, poor sleep, and brain fog.

How can you balance things? Well, first of all, eat regular meals – and definitely don't fast beyond the follicular phase!

Especially important is digging into a blood-sugar loving breakfast within an hour of waking. This will involve some form of protein (aim for at least 25g/¾oz), as well as a portion of healthy fats and complex carbs, if you fancy them.

Keep this up through the day: high protein meals with healthy fats and some complex carbs are where it's at. On top of this, limit any processed and added sugars (artificial sweeteners are doing you no good either!), and add in other blood sugar supportive things, such as going for a walk after meals, drinking a small amount of apple cider vinegar with water before meals, or sprinkling ground cinnamon into foods.

Stuck for meal ideas? Here are some examples of what I eat (although I encourage you to find what works for you, and always consider any allergies you may have):

Breakfast: omelette (two eggs plus two egg whites) with either a sprinkling of cinnamon and nutmeg with berries, dark chocolate, and a scoop of yoghurt, or some feta and veggies. Alternatively, toasted sourdough/homemade bread with scrambled eggs, smoked salmon, and veggies, with a side of berries.

Lunch: last night's leftovers (for example, roast chicken with sweet potatoes), or tinned fish with salad or steamed veggies.

Dinner: grass-fed burger with pickles, homemade wedges and veggies, or homemade bolognese with brown rice pasta.

I often don't need to snack if I've eaten big enough meals, but typical snacks for me if I am hungry include: Greek yoghurt with berries, homemade chocolate cake (recipe in the Winter chapter), or a homemade cacao (recipe in the Autumn chapter), or golden milk (recipe in the Summer chapter) with added collagen or gelatin.

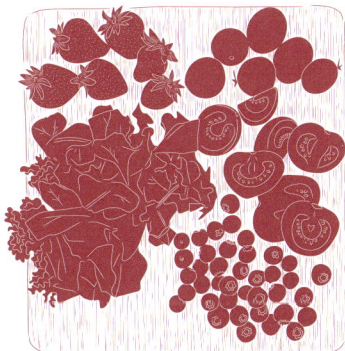

Liver and Gut

The gut and liver play crucial roles in our overall health, but they're especially important for hormones. Signs your gut and liver may need some TLC include acne, bloating, constipation, gas, painful periods, or heavy bleeding. However, if you struggle with persistent bloating, gas, or digestive issues, please get checked out by a doctor to rule out any underlying conditions.

As well as limiting caffeine, alcohol, processed foods, and stress, here are a few of my favourite ways to give these organs some love:

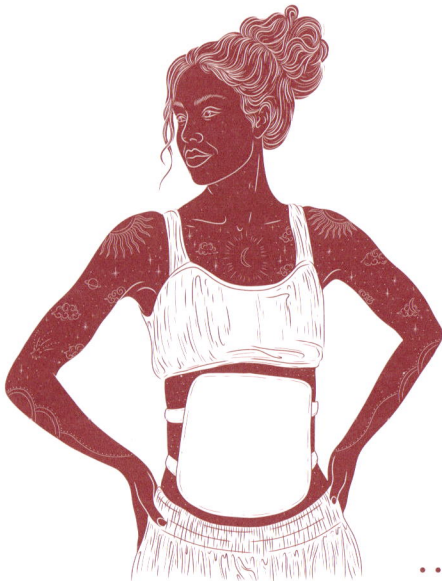

Castor oil packs

Oil-infused wraps to be worn against the skin, castor oil packs are an ancient practice. The oil is known to be powerfully anti-inflammatory and, as well as supporting both liver and gut, it's been linked to shrinking cysts, supporting skin health, boosting healthy digestion, and reducing swelling and pain. However, as a word of caution: don't wear your castor oil pack on your period, which could increase bleeding. There are times (such as during pregnancy, while breastfeeding, and if you are experiencing certain other issues) that castor oil packs shouldn't be used. They also should not be used if you have certain conditions, such as blood disorders or active ulcers. Consult with a medical professional if you are unsure if the packs are suitable for you.

Eating mindfully

How often do you grab a meal on the go, wolfing down food as you race out the door, or hit reply to your 3,002 emails? If you want your gut to be able to digest food properly, you need to eat as mindfully as possible. To do this, signal to your body that you're ready for eating: smell your food, admire it, and even say a small prayer of gratitude. Then, as you eat your meal, try to do it slowly and mindfully, chewing as you go.

Bone broth

Bone broth is another ancient remedy for health, and it works wonders for all kinds of things. However, it's especially good for our gut and our immune system.

Better yet? Bone broth is incredibly cheap to make (often, butchers will give you the bones for free), and tastes delicious. If you can't stomach bone broth, starting your day with a warm lemon water also supports liver health.

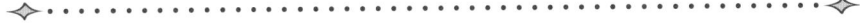

Cruciferous vegetables

Cooked cruciferous vegetables – such as broccoli, cauliflower, and kale – are superfoods for our livers! They help us to flush out excess oestrogen, which ultimately means less PMS. You can try adding them into smoothies (I promise cooked cauliflower is tasteless blended up in a chocolate smoothie!), or making cauliflower or broccoli purée to serve up with grass-fed steak.

Digestive bitters and herbs

If you struggle with bloating, you might like to add digestive bitters to your diet. When eaten at the start of meals, these foods – which include rocket, walnuts, or cacao nibs – support the digestive process. Herbs such as marshmallow root may also be used to help with certain gut issues, but consult with a medical herbalist to find out what's suitable for you.

Detox

Finally, support your body's detox pathways to help flush out toxins. A few ways you can do this include dry body brushing, lymphatic massage sequences (or rebounding), or making sure you get your sweat on regularly – this could be through exercise, but it can equally be found in a hot sauna!

Endocrine Disruptors

Science and medicine are slowly starting to recognise the impact that endocrine disruptors (chemicals that can impact our hormones) may have on our health. Please don't feel you need to be perfect (striving for perfection is not only impossible, but also highly stressful), however here are some things to consider:

· Purchase organic fruit, veg, meat, and dairy wherever possible. If your budget doesn't stretch to this, you can make a homemade wash by soaking produce in filtered water and bicarbonate of soda (1 tsp per 480ml (17oz) of water) for 15 minutes before rinsing. This eliminates up to 90% of pesticides and insecticides.

· Our skin is our largest organ, so consider swapping out toxic make-up or skincare for natural alternatives. I like to use castor oil as a hair mask, tallow as a face moisturiser, and rose-hip oil to nourish skin.

· If you can, avoid using plastics wherever possible, replacing them with alternatives, such as glass bottles or containers.

· Cookware can contain endocrine disruptors, too! Some non-stick pans can be toxic, while aluminium foil may also cause aluminium to leach out into food when heated. If you can afford it, invest in ceramic pots and cast iron pans, and cook using baking paper instead.

· Similarly, consider investing in a good quality water filter. These can be expensive, but they are worth it when you look at the cost-per-use. However, as with anything, please don't stress or get yourself into debt: do the best you can, and buy the best quality you can afford.

Finally, remember that finding joy in life and considering your emotional health matter. If you are in a toxic relationship, surrounded by Energy Vampires, or in a job you loathe or you feel lacks purpose, it will show up in the body in symptoms. The more you love your life, the more you fill it with abundance and love, and the better your health will be.

Epilogue

"When you learn, teach. When you get, give."

Maya Angelou

As you prepare to close this book, I want to take this opportunity to thank you for reading it, and for being such a huge part of my journey. Whether you've read *The Hormone Goddess* cover-to-cover or dipped in and out, I am enormously grateful for you. I love you, and I hope you've found what it is that you needed.

If I could leave you with just one piece of parting advice, sister to sister, it would be to trust in yourself. Listen to your body's inner wisdom, and carve your own path where you need to. There's no "one size fits all". Health comes in all shapes and sizes, and it's about finding what works for you. True health and wellness isn't prescriptive, and it isn't about being perfect.

I hope that you feel more confident in understanding your own body. If you continue to struggle, or if the symptoms of some of the hormonal-related conditions resonated with you, such as PCOS, endometriosis, or thyroid issues, I hope you feel able to seek support. If you feel you're not being taken seriously, please don't be afraid to seek a second opinion. Not all doctors are difficult to deal with (I'd argue that only a minority are), and there are some incredible practitioners out there who are working wonders. You may also find support by working with a nutritional therapist, an alternative practitioner (such as an acupuncturist), or a women's health coach.

Whatever path you tread, please remember to walk with love and compassion. Health and wellness shouldn't feel stressful. The best way (however dull!) is to start with small steps: change one or two things at a time, and build from there. Remember also that healing isn't linear. It's a journey – and, sometimes, it's a long and bumpy one. Even now, my period isn't always perfect. My health isn't always perfect. In fact, as I write this, I've struggled with anxiety over the last few days as my eldest boy prepares to start high school. I've leaned heavily on my toolkit, let myself rest and cry, and done everything I know to regulate my nervous system – and I'm still finding it hard. But, do you know something? That's OK – sometimes, life happens. Stressors happen, traumas happen, our diaries get overloaded, and we bite off more than we can chew. Healing isn't about being perfect, nor is it about never feeling scared, stressed, or anxious again. Instead, true healing is found when we allow ourselves to feel the full rainbow of emotions – and to love and cherish ourselves all the way through them.

if you've found this book helpful, please spread the knowledge far and wide. Pass it on to your sisters, your friends, your daughters, or nieces, and tell any men or boys in your life too! The more people who understand our feminine ebbs and flows, the better. And remember: the more work you do on yourself, the more positive energy, love, and healing will ripple back into the world.

Finally, for all the women who have picked up this book or supported my Instagram page, thank you. Thank you for your outpouring of love, thank you for supporting my work, and thank you for helping me to make a childhood dream come true. But above all, thank you for being part of my own circle of women, of healers, and of walking miracles. You are all my sisters in spirit, and I love you.

Sam xxx

Resources

Organisations

Endometriosis UK
www.endometriosis-uk.org

Endofound (USA)
www.endofound.org

Mind
www.mind.org.uk

Mental Health America
www.mhanational.org

Sane (Australia)
www.sane.org

Practitioners

Emily Nettleton, Medical herbalist
@sulisbotanical on Instagram

Sam Isaacs, Reflexologist
@samjaclynwellbeing on Instagram

Further reading

Cleghorn, Elinor, *Unwell Women: A Journey Through Medicine and Myth in a Man-made World (Weidenfeld & Nicolson, London, 2022)*

Emoto, Masaru, *The Hidden Messages in Water (Simon & Schuster, London, 2005)*

Estes, Clarissa Pinkola, *Women Who Run with the Wolves (Rider, London, 2008)*

Gainsley, Lisa Levitt, *The Book of Lymph (Hodder & Stoughton, London, 2021)*

Northrup, Dr Christiane, *Women's Bodies, Women's Wisdom, 5th edition (Bantam Dell Publishing Group, New York, 2010)*

Owen, Lara, *Her Blood is Gold: Awakening to the Wisdom of Menstruation, 3rd edition (Archive Publishing, Shaftesbury, 2016)*

Shuttle, Penelope and Redgrove, Peter, *The Wise Wound: Menstruation and Everywoman (HarperCollins Publishers, London, 1994)*

About the Author

Sam is a former journalist who retrained as a women's hormone and health coach during the Covid pandemic in 2020. She is also a somatics teacher and womb healer and Priestess. She lives in England with her partner, Amir, and their four boys, plus German Shepherd, Cato. She is at her happiest when she's writing, reading or sat on a beach soaking up the sunshine.

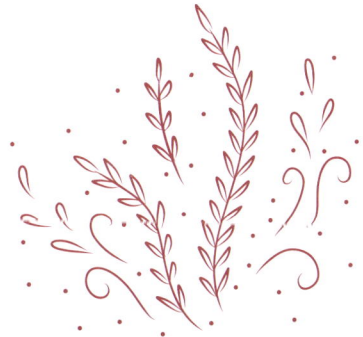

Index

A VERBENA BOOK
© David and Charles, Ltd 2025

Verbena is an imprint of David and Charles,
Ltd, Suite A, Tourism House, Pynes Hill,
Exeter, EX2 5WS

Text © Samantha Hadadi 2025
Layout © David and Charles, Ltd 2025
Illustrations © Irina Chaikova 2025

First published in the UK and USA in 2025

A catalogue record for this book is
available from the British Library.

ISBN-13: 9781446314487 hardback
ISBN-13: 9781446314494 EPUB

This book has been printed on paper from
approved suppliers and made from pulp
from sustainable sources.

FSC
www.fsc.org
MIX
Paper | Supporting
responsible forestry
FSC® C136333

Printed in China through Asia Pacific Offset
for: David and Charles, Ltd, Suite A, Tourism
House, Pynes Hill, Exeter, EX2 5WS

10 9 8 7 6 5 4 3 2 1

Publishing Director: Ame Verso
Senior Commissioning Editor: Lizzie Kaye
Publishing Manager: Jeni Chown
Editor: Victoria Allen
Copy Editor: Jane Trollope
Lead Designer: Sam Staddon
Designer: Lucy Ridley and Lee-May Lim
Pre-press Designer: Susan Reansbury
Illustrations: Irina Chaikova
Production Manager: Beverley Richardson

David and Charles publishes high-quality
books on a wide range of subjects.
For more information visit
www.davidandcharles.com.

Follow us on Instagram by searching for
@dandcbooks.

Layout of the digital edition of this book
may vary depending on reader hardware
and display settings.

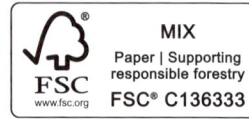

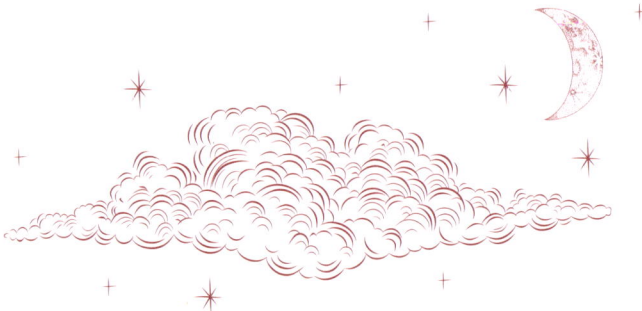

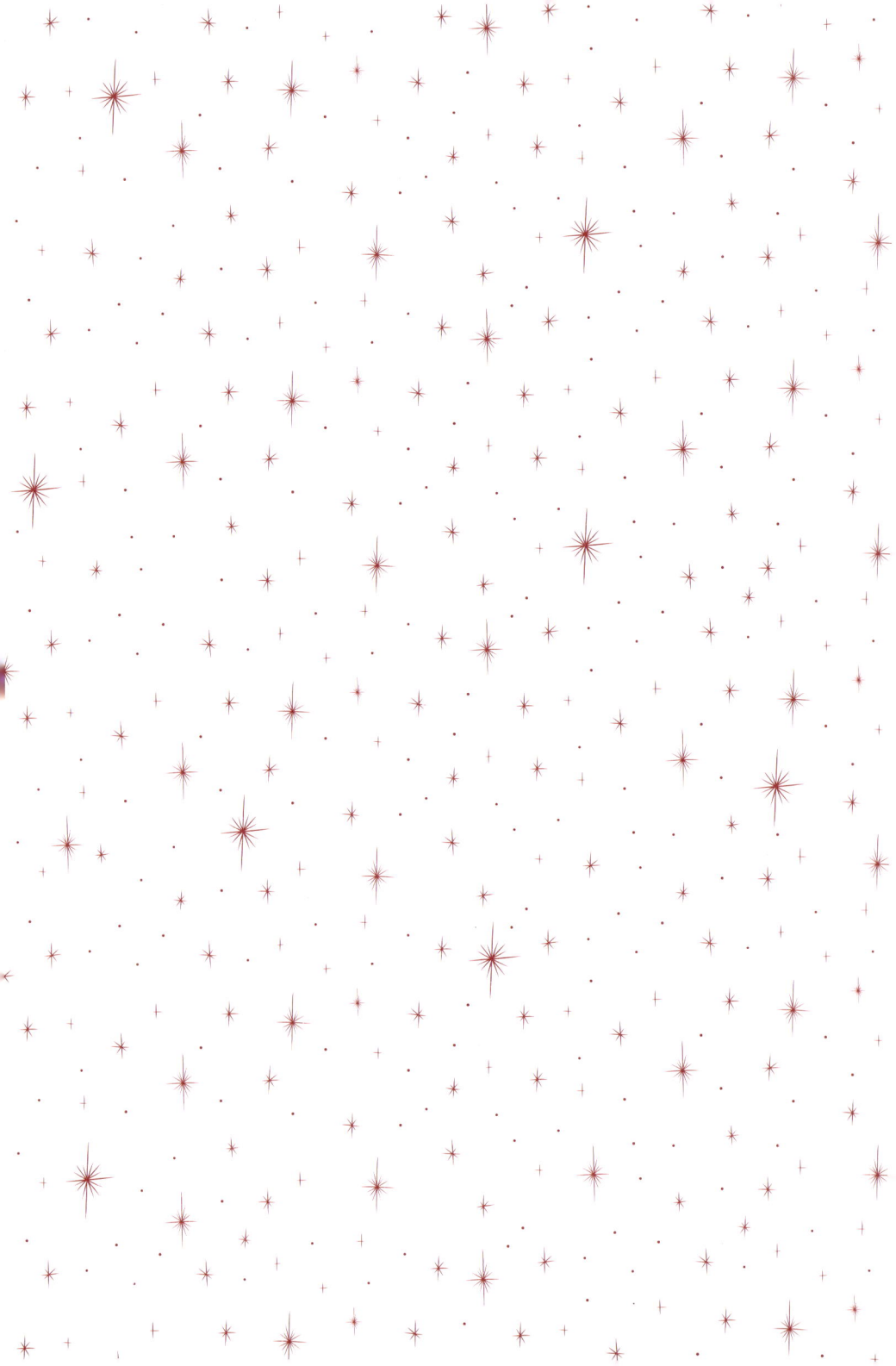